You Can Prevent
And
Reverse Cancer

You Can Prevent

And

Reverse Cancer

Moss Buchanan

Disclaimer: These statements have not been evaluated by the Food and Drug Administration. The products and information contained herein are not intended to diagnose, treat, cure, or prevent any diseases or medical problems. It also is not intended to replace your doctor's recommendations. The information is provided for educational purposes only. Nutritional benefits may vary from one person to another.

This book was printed in the United States of America.

To order additional copies of this book, contact:
Xlibris Corporation
1-888-795-4274
www.Xlibris.com
Orders@Xlibris.com
74317

CONTENTS

To my family and friends.

You are probably not aware, but I made a promise to myself and one to you. I promised I would not let us down and die of cancer. I have overcome one of the greatest obstacles in my life and received many of life's gifts, one of which I would like ever so much to pass on to you.

PROLOGUE

When I was 25 years old, I was 185 cm tall (six feet). I weighed 82 kg (180 lbs). I worked out almost every day and had a physically demanding job in a glass factory. Everyone thought that I was fit. By the time I was 28 years old, I weighed 63 kg (140 lbs) and was in a lot of pain. My family physician told me repeatedly there was nothing wrong with me and that I was fit. A second physician told me the same thing, and to stop wasting his time and good health care dollars. Fortunately, I persisted in my struggle to find out what was wrong with me. That year, I underwent surgery to remove a highly malignant renal cell carcinoma, losing one kidney and one adrenal gland. My prognosis was an eighty percent survival in five years, or a one in five chance of being dead in five years.

The average age for a male to be diagnosed with renal cell carcinoma is over fifty. No one could give me a satisfactory answer as to what caused me at the age of twenty-eight to develop the cancer. No one could give me a satisfactory answer about what I should or should not do to prevent the cancer from coming back. Basically, I was told that I was one of the younger people who had been operated on for such a cancer, and if I survived for five years, then I was "cured". Not good enough!

I took a year to recover to the point that I was able enough to be relatively mobile. Needless to say, I lost my job. However, I continued my studies to acquire my real estate license. But more importantly, I began my search to find satisfactory answers to all the questions that my attending physicians were unable or unwilling to give me. The following is a compendium of my search for some of the answers. Let it be my legacy to all of you that it may help in your fight with cancer.

CHAPTER 1

Background

I thought I was going mad. The answer to cancer seems so simple and obvious to me. It finally came to me when I was forced to take a step back, re-educate myself, and start over from the beginning.

> **Comment:** It was not a schooled electrician who invented the first light bulb. It was not a schooled engineer who invented the first plane. For a long time, the world was flat, and for quite some time, few people would explain how to prevent and reverse cancer.

Let me tell you why I spent so much time thinking and searching for an answer to cancer. I need urgently to tell you this because *I lost four years of my life to cancer.* In fact, I almost lost my whole life to cancer. One year after they removed my tumor, I was still in as much pain as when it started. I have felt the overwhelming fear of not knowing what caused my tumor or how to avoid another one. I have felt the fear of not having the information I require to make myself healthy. I have felt the fear of the grim reaper tapping on my shoulder. I absolutely do not want this to happen to you.

It seems to me that overspecialization in the medical industry has resulted in an inability to see the whole picture. It is becoming more obvious that we cannot just focus on the tumor. Many suggest the body needs to be looked at as a whole. Our bodies are like houses. If one or several pieces of the house are missing, then the whole structure becomes weaker. So I am going to review some of the causes of cancer. I also am going to give you some of the ways to reverse cancer because once you understand cancer, you will realize there are many causes and many ways to reverse it. At the end of this book, you will understand why skinny people and kids get cancer. You are going to understand why we all know someone who smoked their whole life and did not get cancer. You are going to understand why the recurrence rate for chemotherapy is so high. When you put all the pieces together, you are going to understand how you may prevent and reverse cancer. The answer is not a single pill. It is a complex system with many pieces that must all be working together. This is the reason why most cancer remedies have less than 100% success. They rarely address all the weaknesses that have been created in this system. They seem to focus on just one weakness at a time. Each one of these pieces together should create a picture for you. They are what I like to refer to as the building blocks to your house. When all the pieces are in the right place and this picture becomes clear for you, you will be on your way to preventing or reversing cancer.

"New science has pinpointed the cancer answer lies all around you, in your food, your lifestyle, in your environment."

You can prevent cancer. Michael Colgan PhD

CHAPTER 2

How it All Started

When I was a little kid, I always wanted to be a super hero. Funny thing, I always wanted to be Wolverine with his healing powers or Spiderman who always helped others. I know I survived cancer for a reason.

My story begins when I was twenty-eight years old. I had been working rotating shifts as a machine operator for a glass bottle and jar manufacturer for the last three years. I also was taking my real estate courses online in hopes of being self-employed and having more control over my future.

The following is also an important key to understanding the reason I am writing this book. It is the reason I behave and think the way that I do. And, it is the nature of my personality that drives me to pursue this topic in depth. I have an INTP personality. This means Introverted, Intuitive, Thinking, Perceiving, which represents 1 % of the population. The following is how it is applicable.

INTPs have a special gift with generating and analyzing theories and possibilities to prove or disprove them. They have a great deal of insight and are creative thinkers, which allow them to quickly grasp complex abstract thoughts. They also have exceptional logical and rational reasoning skills, which allow them to thoroughly analyze theories to discover the truth about them. Since the INTP is driven to seek clarity in the world, we have a happy match of desire and ability in this personality type.

4http://www.personalitypage.com/INTP_car.html

In school, well-rounded INTPs work on their assignments with a great deal of inward energy and interest that is usually not apparent to others. They tend to connect unrelated thoughts. As learners, they are able to find logical flaws in the thinking of others. They analyze these flaws and find ideas for further study. They go to great depths in their analysis.

INTPs can become obsessed with analysis. Once caught up in a thought process, that thought process seems to have a will of its own for INTPs, and they persevere until the issue is comprehended in all its complexity.

For INTPs, the world exists primarily to be understood. Reality is trivial, a mere arena for proving ideas. It is essential that the universe is understood and that whatever is stated about the universe is stated correctly, with coherence and without redundancy. This is the INTPs final purpose.

http://www.geocities.com/lifexplore/intp.htm

> **Comment:** I already know what I know. I did not write this book for myself. In fact, I would rather not relive this experience at all. This book is being written for you. All of you. Sick or healthy. I hope no one ever has to go through what I went through. Believe me when I tell you, you do not want to go where I have been.

My story begins with lower back pain, groin pain, constant pain and mood swings. All day, all night for months on end. Congratulations to those who managed to put up with me, you are the strong ones. It started with many visits and many complaints about constant lower back and groin pain to my family doctor who after many tests and much effort found nothing. I mean the kind of pain where you cannot stand for more than an hour a day. It was like I had been hit with a sledge hammer in the lower back. Nothing was enjoyable anymore. The kind of pain where all you want to do is sleep and when you wake up, you wish you were asleep again. Never mind the thoughts that were going through my head. My inability to stand forced me to take two months off work and a daily prescription of Percocet. Eventually, I managed to get to the next level of care, specialist number 1 (urologist) who thankfully did many tests, but unfortunately, again found nothing. "Get more exercise. You are young. There is nothing wrong with you." I was told. OK then.

After two months of boredom, I decided to roll myself back into work. At least I would have something else to think about other than the pain. Shortly after returning, one day, I woke up and thought I had pulled a groin muscle because I could not stand up at all. I felt like my left leg was going to fall off. Any movement would cause serious pain to my groin. Back to the doctor. More tests. No hernia. No groin muscle pull. Maybe it was a strain. No answers. Cannot stand up without excruciating pain so I took another two months off work. On to specialist number 2, another urologist. Same complaints, lower backaches, groin pain, constant pain, cannot stand up. More tests. So many tests. Nothing was found. This was frustrating. "Put on more weight," I was told. "And no, you cannot go see another specialist as you have wasted enough health care time already". It is in your head, was the looks I was getting (the same implication that I felt before complaining about migraines). So much pain. Could not work or stand. Could not think straight. Every day was constant agony. Never mind the thoughts in my head. I was about to get fired from work for taking my third two-month break with supposedly no excuse, so the doctor there (at work) sent me to see one of his specialists (an old friend from school) down-town. Almost two years have gone by at this point. I could not believe that I managed to stand up at all. I was running on pure will-power. Every day it was harder to look in the mirror. Those black rings under my eyes were really scaring me. I felt like my life was slipping away quickly.

Fortunately, the attitude was good, and seeing as how so many tests have been done and nothing was found, an MRI was done from my shoulders to my knees. Finally, some resolution! Hurray! Maybe that 2.7 inch tumor in my left kidney was the problem. I assumed it was shock at the time, but it did not seem to scare me too much. As I expected, I was given the option. "Take it out, or you will probably be dead in six months", I was told. I guess you had better sign me up for surgery then. At this point, I was working (somehow) at the plant and taking my real estate courses at the same time. You have to wait for so long to get an exam date, so I pushed my surgery back two days after my phase two (of three) exam.

I will always remember July 27, 2006. Two weeks before my thirtieth birthday. I would rather not talk about the surgery, but I will say it felt like a thick sword had pierced through my body. Imagine pulling a baseball-sized kidney from your lower rib cage to just below your belt and then out through a four-inch incision. I hated the hospital worse than the cemetery. At least in the cemetery, all the pain is gone and it is quiet. Your mind is not trapped in a broken shell. The white walls in the hospital made me feel cold and alone. Oh, and for the nurses out there, a catheter is not supposed to be removed like you are trying to unravel half a roll of toilet paper in one shot. Three years later, I can still notice the effects.

It must have taken me twenty minutes to walk the one hundred feet from my hospital room to the exit of the hospital. The ride home was unbelievable. Even with a good driver, the thought that someone kissing your bumper will kill you is pretty scary. "You will not be able to lift a bag of groceries for six to eight weeks." This, I would soon find out, was a colossal understatement.

I spent the next three months sitting and sleeping in a chair because I could not lie down. I would find out next year, that this is not so great for your back. Insanely bored and super stoned. I was unable to sleep but barely awake. I remember asking to have my tea mugs half full only because I could not lift them up full. I also remember taking my daily walk on my toes for months because the shock of my heels hitting the floor was too much to bear. At the speed I was moving it did not much matter. Two months later, when I did start putting my heels back on the floor it was like walking on a bed of nails. *What is this now?* Terrible needle like sensations in the heel and ball of my foot, which soon after would incur several visits to the doctor, another X-ray and a foot specialist, only to find out that I have now caused heal spurs in my feet that will never (supposedly) go away. Heal spurs can be caused by muscle tension on the bottom of your foot. In its attempt to rebalance, the body grows bone that shortens the distance that the muscle must stretch. The results are small spikes of calcium deposits that micro-tear muscle tissue when you step down. The only solution is to wear foot supports or shoes with a high arch. For those that know me, that is the reason I live in my Adidas Superstars. I had six pairs for a while.

At three months, I told the doctors I was still in pain from the surgery (now taking ten Percs a day barely helping with pain but definitely making me crazy) and I was told that I was still in recovery.

Can anyone tell me the cause of my tumor? Can anyone tell me how to avoid another one? I seem to be healing at lethargic speed. I was going insane with boredom caused by immobility and pain. Same thing at six months, but no one seemed to understand just because I still have the will to move around does not mean that I am not in constant, excruciating pain. I could not sleep on my left side because when I did, it felt like my right kidney was going to drop into the left side of my abdomen. If I sleep on my back somewhere a nerve gets pinched and puts either my arms or legs to sleep. This caused enough sensation to wake me up with pins and needles in my arms every night for the next year. I walked hunched over like a ninety-year old man. Never mind the thoughts in my head. Is it the pain? Could it be the Percs? Doesn't matter, people are counting on me. And why can no one tell me what caused my tumor or how to avoid another one? I have to know. I need to get this question out of my head. This pain is not getting any better. Cancer, cancer, cancer is all I think about, all day, every day. What is going on? I want some answers. And I am going to need them soon.

About six months after my surgery, my sister came back from a two-year trip around the world. I was so excited to see her again I ran (for the first time in ages) down the stairs of my house to catch her at the door. Literally, on the last step, I lost my balance and slipped, only to tear the outside ligament in my left ankle. Sitting on floor, I watched her husband walk away from my front door and missed them both that day. I spent yet another day at the hospital and the next three months on crutches. Still in pain from the surgery, still recovering from the heel spurs, now babysitting a busted ankle. Man, did that hurt. How fortunate I was to have an unlimited supply of Percocet. As I write this book, my ankle still makes a loud popping noise when rotated.

At my one-year visit, I was still complaining about the pain in my groin and lower back, making me unable to stand for more than an hour at a time. The last twenty minutes of the grocery store was always unbearable. I wanted to crawl to my car. One year after surgery and nothing was any better. Three years into a life of constant pain. I felt that my life was slipping away from me at thirty-one. *I want some answers. I won't let you beat me. I refuse to give up.*

Specialist number 4 was supposed to deal with my constant groin pain. After more tests, I was informed that I have varicose veins in my scrotum. Must have developed sometime after my second scrotal ultrasound. Sign me up for procedure number 2. The only suggestion to fix this problem was to insert six—to eight-millimeter platinum coils, launched into my abdomen through a vein, which would then curl up and block some of the network of veins, in hopes of reducing blood flow into my scrotum. I was told they could not put me out, due to the fact I would have to flex at certain points during the procedure. *Oh nice, just what I want, to be awake while a tube was inserted into my neck, through my heart into my abdomen, so you can shoot platinum coils into my body.* Only a one week to recovery, I was told. Not too much pain. Not true. That was not cool. It hurt a lot. Again. The memory of the procedure burns like an emotional scar in my brain. Memories tied to emotion get implanted much deeper in the brain. The only two emotions I could feel at this time were rage and fear. *But I have got to try and keep them hidden, so I can protect those around me.* I needed to stay on the Percs for another two more weeks through the Christmas holidays. January 2008, *So much time has passed. I was starting to feel better. Could this finally be the end of the pain?*

By the way, at this point, I still have not told my sister or my mother about my cancer. In the beginning, I did not want to tell my sister by e-mail or have her come back from her trip because of me. I did not want my mom to suffer the emotional trauma that moms suffer when their child is hurt. My plan was to get better first, and then I would tell them. All they would have done is worry. Unfortunately, that was not going to help me.

January was great, and so was the start of February. It seemed like I was starting to get better. After two years or so of Percocets, my mind was getting a little foggy to say the least. It would have been nice if anyone of the many doctors I had visited could have told me not to forget to wean myself off the pills. But I did forget. I wanted so badly to have my brain back that I just stopped—cold turkey. Went from two Percs every four hours to none at all in one day. Seemed okay. My willpower and motivation are very strong. However, a few weeks later, I started to notice the withdrawal symptoms. Oh wow, did I ever! I would feel hot then cold. Happy, then painfully sad. Then very, very angry with a little bit of suicidal thoughts mixed in. The shakes came often. All my nerve endings felt sensitive as feeling started to return to my body. Unclear, broken thoughts about cancer and what I had just done to myself were floating around in my head all day. I was afraid to go outside of my house for fear of what I might do to anyone who did as little as say "Hi" to me. *I can beat this. Failure is not an option. This is, what should be, the last hurtle of my recovery.* But as you may have expected, the story does not end here.

Shortly after the withdrawal symptoms started to fade away, I noticed this small fireball of pain about five inches up my rectum. Enough to cause random lightning bolts of searing pain that knocked me to the floor on five different occasions. Imagine an unexpected lightning bolt of pain so forceful it knocks you to your knees. Not cool. You have to be kidding me! Back to Specialist number 4. Oh yay, more pills. Prostate infection was the diagnosis. A month on the highest dose of antibiotics available. The $190 worth of pills made me sicker than I have ever felt in my entire life. I could not move. My body was so stiff my blood felt like hard syrup. I experienced the most severe full-body cramping of my life. It felt like my whole body was being crushed in a vice. Dizziness came and went. I could not think straight. I felt like I was in a half-coma state fifteen hours a day. My body felt like it was turning to stone. I could barely muster enough energy to crawl to washroom. *I have been in agony for over two years, and NOW I think I just might be ready to let go. The mind can only take so much. I have been pushing maximum for a long while now.* "Just keeping taking the pills," I was told about ten days in. Week two I took myself off them. *As high as I am, something does not add up. Nothing the doctors have done so far has relieved any pain. How can it get any worse?*

I did not stop searching for answers though. I went right back and asked them what is next. I will tell you how it can get worse. This is the thing that scared me the most. Like a cocked gun being held in your face by a masked man. Even scarier than being told I had cancer. The next stop for me was permanent pain killers (I am guessing man-made pharmaceuticals) at the pain clinic downtown. All I heard was, "We have no more answers for you, young man. You are going to die. We will try to dull your pain for the rest of your time here." That was the crushing blow I needed. I could not take it anymore. Failure was never an option. I knew it was time to deviate from Western medicine and search for an alternative therapy.

I am glad I did. I am completely positive that it is the only reason I am alive today.

I can not move around. I can not sleep. Might as well read. I will not let you beat me. Too many people are counting on me to get better. I refuse to give up. I have come too far now. I will not quit. Seven days a week for the next year and a half straight, between eight and eighteen hours a day, all I did was read. There are only a few books on cancer at the bookstore, so I spent most of my time on the Internet. All day, all night. *Read about the human body. Search for answers. Put the pieces together. Someone knows the answer to this question, but who?*

Two days before my two-year surgery celebration, I had an epiphany.

It was when I developed the simple understanding that *we all have cancer cells in our body.* Supposedly millions throughout a lifetime according to Sir Peter Medawar. *When the body is healthy, they are destroyed without any difficulty . . .*

US Research Report #100: Adjuvant Nutrition for Cancer Patients, Jan 15, 1993.

Hmmm, what does this mean?

We are all cancer patients! Unfortunately, some of us have let our cancer get out of control or balance as I think it can be referred to since cancer cells or cellular deviations are unavoidable.

> **Comment:** If cancer has developed inside you, then you and your cancer are as one. I am merely suggesting this is how the problem should be looked at—as a whole. If you were to get a cold and start coughing, it would make no sense to take your lungs out, part of your throat, and possibly your nose. Just because a part of your body gets sick does not mean that you should cut it out. What needs to be done is to *address the problem* and return the body to a state of balance. Every part of the body must be working properly for

optimum health and healing. It is kind of like an arch. If any small piece of the arch is missing, then the whole thing will get weak and start to collapse. You do not have to understand exactly how all the pieces of the arch work *per se*, you just need to remember that they all have to be there. When they are all there, they will all be working together to keep your body healthy, like the pieces of an arch.

All cancers begin in cells, the body's basic units of life. To understand cancer, it is helpful to know what happens when normal cells become cancer cells.

The body is made up of many types of cells. These cells grow and divide in a controlled way to produce more cells as they are needed to keep the body healthy. When cells become old or damaged, they die and are replaced with new cells.

However, sometimes this orderly process goes wrong. The genetic material (DNA) of a cell can become damaged or changed, producing mutations that affect normal cell growth and division. When this happens, cells do not die when they should and new cells form when the body does not need them. The extra cells may form a mass of tissue called a tumor.

http://www.cancer.gov/cancertopics/what-is-cancer

> **Comment:** Cancer tumors are caused by DNA mistakes. The way to avoid these mistakes getting out of control is to facilitate a healthy body. This book represents a three-year evolution of a system that has been designed to facilitate a very healthy body, because when you have a healthy body, cancer cannot survive.

CHAPTER 3

Why They Don't Want You to Know

"If you want to manipulate people, it is essential that you have knowledge that they don't have."

Unknown

> **Comment:** This is the reason why many doctors will disagree with some of the ideas that I present to you. They do not have the same information. What we need to ask ourselves is, why? Why do they appear not to have this information? And better yet, why is this information not being better researched? The results always tell the real truth. The results are cancer is more rampant than ever. The real truth is that the pharmaceutical industry is one of the largest industries in the world, and you are worth nothing healthy.

> **Comment:** Information is being suppressed in the interest of profits. This has been true since the dawn of time. And now, the medical industry has made it illegal for anyone other than a medical doctor to use the word *drug* or *cure*. Nobody else other than a medical doctor can diagnose, treat, or prescribe something to cure you. I cannot say water is the *cure* for dehydration. And therefore, no one can ever legally say a vitamin or a herb is a *cure* for anything. Even though most drugs are made from derivatives of herbs! Ask yourself, What is the purpose of this? Why would the medical industry not want any herb or natural remedy (that cannot be patented) to be considered a *cure*?

> **Comment:** Less than 2% of money donated to cancer research goes towards natural remedies. The other 98% goes towards making pharmaceutical drugs that will be sold back to you for thousands of dollars per dose. People are *paying* to stay alive.

"There will never be a CURE for Cancer until the Establishment can accomplish their objectives by permitting it."

Dr Kelley DDS

> **Comment:** If the answer comes out and people live longer, what will happen to the supposedly already too large world population? Or the billions of dollars made annually by cancer research, operations, and drugs? Could that be the reason that less than 2% of the money that goes to cancer research is spent on natural cures that would incur little or no profit?

"It is estimated that if people had a choice, lack of demand would shrink Doctors and Drugs to less than 10% of its current size, with the remainder almost entirely related to trauma medicine. That would be a $ 900,000,000,000.00 (nine hundred BILLION dollar) loss to them. They are not going to take this loss without a good fight."

Dr Shulze

> **Comment:** Much of my research started from a list I have (two pages long) of doctors who say that they understand cancer and have a method of reversing it. Each one of them has either been killed in a car accident, been mysteriously poisoned or committed an unexplained suicide.

"Every discoverer of a cancer remedy has encountered a Chinese wall of resistance, which has been the same in every page of recorded cancer history, and that the myth that the discoverer of a cancer cure would be "honored, acclaimed, and practically deified as a savior of the human race," should be changed to "dishonored, denounced and crucified, unless he is a fair haired boy of the dominating oligarchy."

The Cancer Blackout: An Illuminating, Factual Survey by M. H. Clutter, D.R.L

> **Comment:** This was not easy to find.

Georgia's informed consent law requires physicians, before performing surgery, to inform their patients of the risks and of "practical alternatives . . . *which are generally recognized and accepted* by reasonably prudent physicians."

UNITED STATES DISTRICT COURT
SOUTHERN DISTRICT OF GEORGIA, BRUNSWICK DIVISION

Comment: Does this not mean you will only recommend what you learned in school? I.e., what is the most beneficial for *your* business as opposed to what is in my best interest? If this is the case, are we not being shorted some possible answers? Is the 5% of time spent on nutrition at Harvard Medical School enough? The earth was absolutely flat for quite some time. Then it became round. Or was it always round?

Comment: In China, cancer is considered little more than a bad cold. It is considered reversible under the correct conditions. However, if you knew what the correct conditions were, you would be of lesser value to the multi billion dollar medical and pharmaceutical industry.

According to some, more than 7.5 million unnecessary medical and surgical procedures are performed annually. The number of people exposed to unnecessary hospitalization annually is 8.9 million. Even more frightening is the fact that the American medical system is the leading cause of death and injury in the United States! Meanwhile, the pharmaceutical industry's profits last year hit $377 billion!

http://t.webring.com/hub?ring=naturalcuresthey

Comment: The Canadian government has just been frowned upon for investing pension money in tobacco. Yet they spend money (your tax money) on "quit smoking" campaigns. Is this not a contradiction? The same government is trying to tell us that cigarettes being behind a metal curtain will stop kids from smoking. In marketing (or politics), we call this misdirection. A rule put in place only to appease the public. Are they really looking after "your best interests"? Or are they only interested in money?

I suggest to you that the reason they do not want you to know is money.

CHAPTER 4

Oncogenes and Tumor-Suppressor Genes

Comment: First we need to remember that everything we know of begins with atoms. Atoms make up molecules that make up cell structures or extracellular components, and these structures make up cells, which make up tissues, which make up organs. But, it all begins with atoms.

Each atom has a nucleus and protons in the center. On the outer shell of the atom are electron (see diagram next page).

Inside the nucleus of each atom is a "mapping system" known as DNA. DNA is a vast chemical information database that carries the complete set of instructions for making all the proteins a cell will ever need.

This DNA "mapping system" is made up of subunits called "genes". A gene is any given segment along the DNA that encodes instructions that allow a cell to produce a specific product, typically, a protein such as an enzyme that initiates one specific action. For example: the division speed or growth rate of a cell. (Both of these actions, if not instructed properly, could potentially cause cancer).

http://rarediseases.about.com/od/geneticdisorders/a/genesbasics.htm

http://www.accessexcellence.org/AE/AEPC/NIH/gene03.php

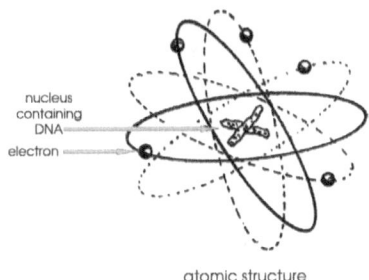

atomic structure

Comment: Within this DNA "mapping system", there are two types of genes that are commonly discussed when speaking about cancer. The first are oncogenes, and the second are tumor-suppressor genes.

Oncogenes: Inside the nucleus of most cells in the body, there are hundreds of thousands of genes. Each gene is made up of a specific DNA sequence that contains the code (the instructions) for that gene's function. Oncogenes, on the other hand, are mutations of a normal gene (originally called a proto-oncogene). When this occurs, part of the DNA "mapping system" is damaged, and the result is an oncogene (bad) that may be permanently turned on when it is not supposed to be. For example, if the gene or "switch" for growth is turned on and runs out of control, this can lead to cancer. Most oncogenes are acquired; however, 5 to 10% are hereditary (from your parents at birth). This may mean you have a higher risk of cancer, but it does not mean that you cannot do anything to fight it.

http://www.cancer.org/docroot/eto/content/eto_1_4x_oncogenes_and_tumor_suppressor_genes.asp

Comment: The other types of genes that can cause cancer are "tumor-suppressor genes". They can be thought of as an "off" switch for cancer. If the "off" switch breaks or is turned on, then cancer will begin to grow out of control.

Tumor-suppressor genes are normal genes that slow down cell division, repair DNA mistakes, and tell cells when to die (a process known as *apoptosis* or *programmed cell death*). When tumor suppressor genes do not work properly, cells can grow out of control, which can lead to cancer.

http://www.cancer.org/docroot/eto/content/eto_1_4x_oncogenes_and_tumor_suppressor_genes.asp

Comment: Genes tell the cell what to do. Sometimes genes say *"go"*, and sometimes they say *"stop"*. However, if this part of the DNA "mapping system" does not function properly, cells can grow out of control and possibly cause cancer.

CHAPTER 5

How Viruses Can Cause Cancer

Comment: Viruses are made up of a small group of genes surrounded by a protein coating. They cannot reproduce on their own, so they function by attaching to another host cell. After attaching, viruses inject their own DNA (or RNA), which can disrupt the original DNA sequence of the "host" cell. This disruption of the original DNA sequence (or mapping system) may cause a cell to become cancerous. However, this does not mean that every virus you acquire will cause cancer. Most will cause only a very minimal disruption to the cellular "mapping system" (DNA) and therefore to your body. Conversely, some viruses can, if they affect the right gene(s), cause cancer.

http://www.cancer.org/docroot/PED/content/PED_1_3X_Infectious_Agents_and_Cancer.asp

Viruses Linked to Cancer:

1. Cervical cancer, and other cancers of the genital and anal area, and the genital wart
2. Virus, HPV primary liver cancer, and the Hepatitis B and C viruses
3. Lymphomas and the Epstein-Barr virus
4. T-cell leukemia in adults and the human T-cell leukemia virus
   HPV also probably leads to oropharyngeal cancer and non-melanoma skin cancers in some people

   Comment: In conclusion, all you really need to understand is that cancer is caused by mistakes or changes in the DNA "mapping system". This can cause cells to grow out of control, which is cancer. This damage can occur in several ways such as hereditary mistakes, gene mutations (oncogenes), viruses, or free radicals, which we will discuss in the next chapter.

http://www.cancerhelp.org.uk/about-cancer/causes-symptoms/causes/what-causes-cancer

CHAPTER 6

Understanding Free Radicals (Electron Thieves)

Comment: This is the second step towards understanding cancer. This is usually how a cancer tumor first begins. I like to think of the body as a house that requires many pieces to be complete. Free radicals, to me, are kind of like having "termites" in your house. They run around and "steal" electrons, which can potentially damage vital pieces of your DNA, which, as we know, is the "mapping system" to the cells in our bodies. How well can we be expected to build something complicated without the right set of instructions?

Cancer begins in your body every day with a free radical damaging a single atom by stealing an electron (unless your cancer is caused by a virus or an oncogene). If this problem is not repaired quickly (preferably with an antioxidant) this chain of destruction will continue.

Free radicals are highly reactive atoms or groups of atoms with an odd (unpaired) number of electrons, which in an attempt to maintain a stable structure, "steal" their missing electron from another molecule. When the "attacked" molecule loses *its* electron, it becomes a free radical itself (*unstable* atom missing an electron), thus, beginning a negative chain reaction.

http://www.healthchecksystems.com/antioxid.htm

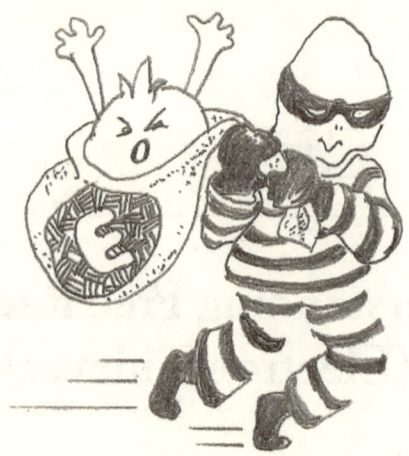

Free radicals steal electrons

How Free Radicals Are Formed: The Basics

Comment: Normally, bonds do not split in a way that leaves a molecule with an odd, unpaired electron. But when weak bonds split, free radicals are formed. Free radicals are very unstable and react quickly with other compounds, *trying to capture the needed electron to gain stability.* Generally, free radicals attack the nearest stable molecule, "stealing" its electron. As previously stated, when the "attacked" molecule loses its electron, it becomes a free radical itself, beginning a chain reaction. Once the process is started, it can cascade, finally resulting in the disruption of a living cell.

Comment: Acidity means a 'low pH', which, in turn, can be classified as an excess of protons and *a lack of electrons.* Atoms missing an electron (acidic) are destructive. (This will be discussed in later chapters on pH levels and ionized water.)

Comment: Antioxidants are one of the things that maintain "balance" with the free radicals in our bodies. They run around the body saying, "Hey, are there any free radicals missing an electron, because I have an extra one to give away?"

Antioxidants neutralize free radicals by "*donating* one of their own electrons", ending the electron "stealing" reaction. The antioxidant nutrients themselves do not become free radicals by donating an electron because they are stable in either form. They act as scavengers, helping to prevent cell and tissue damage that could lead to cellular damage and disease.

http://www.healthchecksystems.com/antioxid.htm

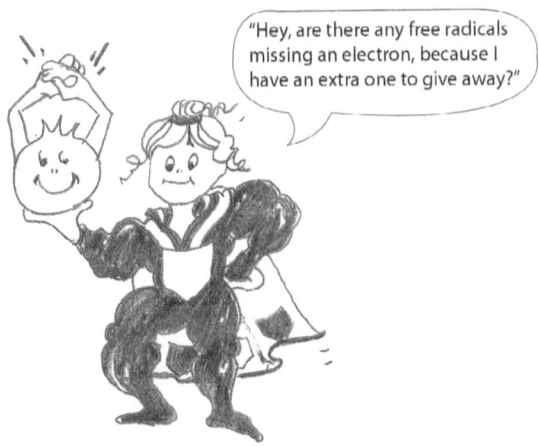

"Hey, are there any free radicals missing an electron, because I have an extra one to give away?"

How might antioxidants prevent cancer? Antioxidants neutralize free radicals as the natural by-product of normal cell processes. Free radicals are molecules with incomplete electron shells, which make them more chemically reactive than those with complete electron shells. Exposure to various environmental factors, including tobacco smoke and radiation, can also lead to free radical formation. In humans, the most common form of free radicals is oxygen. When an oxygen molecule (O_2) becomes electrically charged or "radicalized", it tries to steal electrons from other molecules, causing damage to the DNA and other molecules. Over time, such damage may become irreversible and lead to disease including cancer. Antioxidants are often described as "mopping-up" free radicals, meaning they neutralize the electrical charge and prevent the free radical from taking electrons from other molecules.

1. Blot WJ, Li JY, Taylor PR et al. Nutrition intervention trials in Linxian, China: supplementation with specific vitamin/mineral combinations, cancer incidence, and disease-specific mortality in the general population. J Natl Cancer Inst 1993; 85:1483-91.
2. The Alpha-Tocopherol, Beta Carotene Cancer Prevention Study Group. The effects of vitamin E and beta carotene on the incidence of lung cancer and other cancers in male smokers. N Engl J Med 1994; 330:1029-35.
3. Omenn GS, Goodman G, Thomquist M et al. The beta-carotene and retinol efficacy trial (CARET) for chemo prevention of lung cancer in

high risk populations: smokers and asbestos-exposed workers. Cancer Res 1994; 54(7 Suppl):2038s-43s.

4. Hennekens CH, Buring JE, Manson JE et al. Lack of effect of long-term supplementation with beta carotene on the incidence of malignant neoplasms and cardiovascular disease. N Engl J Med 1996; 334:1145-9.

5. Lee IM, Cook NR, Manson JE. Beta-carotene supplementation and incidence of cancer and cardiovascular disease: Women's Health Study. J Natl Cancer Inst 1999; 91:2102-6.

http://www.cancer.gov/cancertopics/factsheet/antioxidantsprevention

Comment: So in order to deal with cancer, we need to understand that free radicals and antioxidants must be balanced (so as not to damage the DNA "mapping system"). If you have too many destructive free radicals in your body, it will break itself down at a high rate of speed. If you have too many antioxidants, it will cause other problems including reductive stress and start to make you sick as well. Your body, with all of its daily functions, is producing free radicals constantly, so it is imperative to make sure you are getting antioxidants in your diet. That being said, overdosing on antioxidants with a regular diet and exercise is extremely difficult. However, I have done this on one occasion in the last two years, so I know personally that it can be done. Balancing the two is the key.

Unfortunately, there is much more to understand when battling cancer than just how free radicals steal electrons and potentially cause damage to the DNA "mapping system". As I stated before, there are many pieces to this house that is your body. Just like the pieces of an "arch," they must all be working together in order for your body to function and heal properly. When your body is functioning and healing properly, cancer cannot survive.

CHAPTER 7

Immune System: Your Last Defense

Comment: Part of the final battle against cancer, your immune system seeks out things that do not belong and destroys them (like cancer cells and viruses). If it does not work, then you can not even fight your basic cold. Your immune system is sort of like having a full-time butler that cleans up all the messes that occur in your house (like cancer cells). Conversely, if he is not taken care of or is overworked, he will get upset and destroy things that he is supposed to clean (autoimmune disease). Your immune system is a critical piece of the equation that must be considered when preventing or reversing cancer.

Cancerous cells are *always* being created in the body. Consequently, there are parts of your immune system that are designed to seek out and destroy cancer cells. Cancer has been around as long as mankind, but only in the second half of the twentieth century did the number of cancer cases explode. Contributing to this explosion are the excessive amounts of toxins and pollutants to which we are constantly being exposed; for example, high stress lifestyles that deplete the immune system, poor quality junk food that is full of pesticides, electromagnetic stress (see chapter on EMFs), low-quality air, fluorinated water (see chapter on fluoride) or just about everything that was not here one hundred years ago. All these things *weaken* your immune system, thereby promoting the growth of cancer.

Cancer is *not* a mysterious disease that suddenly attacks you out of the blue. It has definite causes that *you can correct* if your body has enough time, and if you *take action now* to change the internal environment to one that facilitates good health, not cancer. Cancer tumors begin when more cancerous cells are being created than your immune system can destroy. For most of your life, your immune system has successfully dealt with cancer cells, killing them off as they developed. For cancer to have developed in you, your immune system must have become worn-out, ineffective, or unable to deal with the cancer cells.

Because of this stress and the overload of toxins, you end up with a malfunctioning immune system and a body that is *not* capable of destroying the excessive number of cancerous cells that develop. Some survive, multiply, and then you have cancer. Overcoming cancer is a process of *reversing* the conditions that allowed the cancer to develop. *Going after and killing cancerous cells.* The exact causes do not have to be known though certainly the more varied the approaches taken, the more likely you are going to hit on what works best for you. What you need to do is to strongly and dramatically interrupt and reverse the cancer-causing conditions in your body so that your body becomes healthier and stops breeding cancer.

Note: Chemotherapy, which costs 50 to 250 thousand dollars per treatment, *damages all cells* and weakens the immune system. You also should know that recommending "natural or alternative health therapies" is against hospital insurance regulations. Advice is controlled by a large medical industry, an industry that does not look favorably on natural supplements or other cancer treatments. Interestingly, these treatments cannot be patented to make high profits.

http://www.cancerfightingstrategies.com/index.html

Things That Can Go Wrong With the Immune System

Disorders of the immune system can be broken down into four main categories:

1. immunodeficiency disorders (primary or acquired).
2. autoimmune disorders (in which the body's own immune system attacks its own tissue as foreign matter). I suggest this is caused by an overdose of "junk" in the body—so much clutter in the house the butler does not even know what to clean anymore.
3. allergic disorders (in which the immune system overreacts in response to an antigen).
4. cancers of the immune system.

Cancers of the Immune System

Cancer occurs when cells grow out of control. This can also happen with the cells of the immune system. Lymphoma involves the lymphoid tissues and is one of the more common childhood cancers. Leukemia, which involves abnormal overgrowth of leukocytes, is the most common childhood cancer.

With current medications, most cases of both types of cancer in kids and teens are curable.

http://kidshealth.org/parent/general/body_basics/immune.html

Tumors are merely one of the symptoms of an underlying systemic disease. Shrinkage or even disappearance of tumors *still leaves the disease intact.* That may be why so many cancers reoccur.

You can prevent cancer. Michael Colgan, PhD

> **Comment:** I suggest that this is the reason why I did not get any better after my kidney was removed. My surgery did not ameliorate the underlying causes of my sickness, one of which being a weakened immune system.

When normal cells mutate into cancer cells, some of the antigens on their surface change. These cells, like many body cells, constantly shed bits of protein from their surface into the circulatory system. Often, tumor antigens are among the shed proteins.

These shed antigens prompt action from immune defenders, including cytotoxic T cells, natural killer cells, and macrophages. According to one theory, patrolling cells of the immune system provide continuous body-wide surveillance, catching and eliminating cells that undergo malignant transformation. Tumors develop when this immune surveillance breaks down or is overwhelmed.

http://www.cancer.gov/cancertopics/understandingcancer/immunesystem/Slide32

Although the immune system can recognize viral strains it has encountered and beaten off before, it will not recognize a virus that has mutated, and even the smallest genetic change will trick the immune system into thinking a brand new species, for which it has no antibodies, has landed. While a strong immune system will cope with this attack, one that has been weakened by poor nutrition and too much stress will struggle to get you back to good health.

> **Comment:** Why do I take antibiotics for a cold (viral infection) when I could take natural immune system boosters (such as colostrum or astragalus) and natural virus killers (such as oregano oil)? Slow wound healing, repeated infections, fatigue, colds, flu, and allergies

are all signs that the body's immune system is functioning below par. As healthy adults, we should suffer no more than two colds per year. If you are getting sicker for longer with every passing infection, you definitely need to start supporting your immune system.

Comment: Consider this next article for a moment, if you will.

When something dies, its immune system (along with everything else) shuts down. *In a matter of hours*, the body is invaded by all sorts of bacteria, microbes, parasites. None of these things are able to get in when your immune system is working, but the moment your immune system stops, the door is wide open. Once you die, it only takes a few weeks for these organisms to completely dismantle your body and carry it away, until all that is left is a skeleton. Obviously, your immune system is doing something amazing to keep all of that dismantling from happening when you are alive.

http://www.howstuffworks.com/immune-system.htm

Comment: Your immune system attacks things it does not like in your body. For you to fight cancer or just be healthy, your immune system must be functioning properly. Sadly, for it to function properly, the other "pieces" of this equation or "arch" must be functioning properly as well.

CHAPTER 8

How pH Levels Affect Cancer

Comment: So we have discussed how genes go awry. We have reviewed how free radicals and antioxidants play together. We have looked at the role of the immune system. All these "pieces" must work together like a team, and to work effectively, they must do so in an ambient environment. Thus, we must consider next our pH level. The pH level in your body is kind of like the thermostat in your house. If it goes too low (acidic) or too high (alkaline), there will be a major disruption in the activities that go on inside. The key is balance. The ideal blood pH is around 7.45, which is neutral. I am positive that an acidic pH contributed to a large part of my cancer problem, simply because I had been eating acidic foods with little nutritional value since the time when I moved out on my own fifteen years ago.

"The doctor of the future will give no medicine, but will interest his patients in the care of the human frame, in diet, and in the cause and prevention of disease."

Thomas A. Edison

What Most People Don't Realize: We Are Bioelectrical Engines

In order to accomplish all the many millions of complex functions that occur over the course of the day, your body has to be able to communicate with itself all the way down to the cellular level. And do you know how it does this? Through pulses of electricity. That is right—electricity.

Your body operates on an electromagnetic current. Believe it or not, all of the organs in your body emit these fields of electrical current. In fact, nerve signals are nothing more than electrical charges.

> **Comment:** According to my acupuncture doctor, a muscle twitch is "a block in chi flow" or "energy". I have experienced this sensation, and I believe he is correct.

What creates this electrical power in your body is a very fine balance that exists in your biochemistry. And of all the systems in your body that depend on this delicate, biochemical balance, one of the most important is your bloodstream. This is where pH comes into play. But what is pH?

PH is a scale that measures how acidic or alkaline a substance is. The scale ranges from 1 to 14 with 1 being very acid, 7 neutral, and 14 very alkaline. If blood pH moves below 6.8 or above 7.8, cells stop functioning, and the body dies.

http://www.trans4mind.com/nutrition/pH.html

So what does pH have to do with you and your blood? Well, the pH of your blood is extremely important. The ideal pH level for your blood is right *around* 7.45, and your body goes to enormous lengths to maintain this level.

Why? Because if your blood pH were to vary by even a few points in either direction, it would change the electrical chemistry in your body. There would be no electrical power and in short order, you would drop dead. As you can see, maintaining the right pH level in your blood is pretty important.

With this in mind, a good way to avoid upsetting this delicate biochemical balance would be to take a look at those things that can compromise the maintenance of the ideal pH level in your body. And what is the main culprit in this case? The answer is the creation of acid in your body.

Red blood cells transport oxygen to all the cells in your body. As red blood cells move into the tiny, capillaries, the space they have to move through gets pretty small. In fact, the diameter of the capillaries gets so small that the red blood cells sometimes have to pass through these capillaries one red blood cell at a time!

Because of this, and because it is important for the red blood cells to be able to flow easily and quickly through your body, they have a mechanism that allows them to remain separate from each other. This mechanism comes in the form of the outside of healthy red blood cells having a negative charge. This causes them to stay apart from each other, sort of like when you try to push the negative ends of two magnets together. They resist each other and stay apart.

Unfortunately, acid interferes with this very important mechanism in a pretty frightening way. Acid actually strips away the negative charge from red blood cells. The result is that your red blood cells then tend to clump together and not flow as easily. This makes it much more difficult for them to flow easily through the bloodstream.

But it also makes it harder for them to move freely through those small capillaries. This means less oxygen gets to your cells. Acid also weakens the red blood cells, and they begin to die. And guess what they release into your system when they die? More acid.

In regard to producing energy in the body, here is an easy question for you. What do you think happens to a person's energy level if over time their system becomes more and more acidic, their biochemical balance is disrupted, and their red blood cells can not deliver oxygen and nutrients as efficiently to all their cells? The answer is simple. Their energy level drops. Dramatically.

According to Keiichi Morishita, in his book *Hidden Truth of Cancer*, when your blood starts to become acidic, your body deposits acidic substances in the blood (usually toxins) into cells to allow the blood to remain slightly alkaline. However, this causes your cells to become more acidic and toxic, which results in a decrease of their oxygen levels, which, in turn harms their DNA and respiratory enzymes.

Over time, he theorizes, these cells increase in acidity, and some die. These dead cells themselves turn into acids. However, *some* of these acidified cells may *adapt* in that environment. In other words, instead of dying (as normal cells do in an acid environment), some cells survive by becoming abnormal cells.

These abnormal cells are called malignant cells. Malignant cells do not correspond with brain function nor with our own DNA memory code. Therefore, malignant cells grow indefinitely and without order. This is cancer.

http://www.cancerfightingstrategies.com/acidity.html

What Causes Acid in the Body

The primary cause of an acidic condition in your body is from what you put in your mouth. In other words, what you eat and what you drink. And it is not how "acidic" something may seem when you eat or drink it. It has to do with what is left over after you digest it.

Specifically, eating or drinking something results in the formation of an acid or alkaline "ash". For example, when your body digests scallops, it leaves an extremely acid ash. In fact, scallops are one of the most acid foods you can eat.

There is plenty of research showing that cancer thrives in an acidic environment and does not survive in a normal, more alkaline environment. Cancer cells make your body even more acidic as they produce lactic acid. So if you have cancer, your pH levels are low, and your body is too acidic.

Alkaline water (including the water in cells) holds a lot of oxygen. Acidic water holds very little oxygen. So the more acidic your cells are, the less oxygenated they will be. To make matters worse, the fermentation process cancer cells use to produce energy creates lactic acid, further increasing acidity and reducing oxygen levels (see chapter on ionized water).

Sang Whang, in his book *Reverse Aging*, points out that toxins are acidic. If your blood is too acidic, toxins will not be released from your cells into the blood. So your cells can not be detoxified. This buildup of toxins in your cells results in acidic, poorly oxygenated cells, which can turn cancerous. He explains,

"In general, degenerative diseases are the result of acid waste buildups within us. When we are born, we have the highest alkaline mineral concentration and also the highest body pH. From that point on, the normal process of life is to gradually acidify. That is why these degenerative diseases do not occur when you are young. Reverse aging requires two separate steps: chemical and physical. The first step is to lower the acidity of the body so that it can dispose of acidic wastes in the blood and cellular fluids safely and easily. The second step is to physically pull out old stored wastes into the blood stream so that they can be discharged from the body."

There is a long history of reversing cancer simply by alkalinizing the body. It is one of the basic strategies in the battle against cancer and for improving your health in general.

Virtually everyone with cancer has low pH levels.

http://www.cancerfightingstrategies.com/acidity.html

> **Comment:** It is helpful to remember that things that are in an acidic state have an "unbalanced" electron. Due to this imbalance, these acidic atoms will damage and disrupt anything they come into contact with. The inverse is also true. Things in an alkaline state have a spare or "extra" electron and, as such, will be more than happy to share or give the extra electron up to those in need.

Unfortunately, a lot of the things most people put in their mouths create an acid ash. These include meats, alcohol, grains, sugar and coffee. Interestingly enough, *stress* also tends to create an acid condition in the body.

An imbalanced diet high in acidic-producing foods such as animal protein, sugar, caffeine, and processed foods puts pressure on the body's regulating systems to maintain pH neutrality. The extra buffering required can deplete the body of alkaline minerals such as sodium, potassium, magnesium, and calcium, making the person prone to chronic and degenerative disease. Minerals are borrowed from vital organs and bones to buffer (neutralize) the acid and safely remove it from the body. Because of this strain, the body can suffer severe and prolonged damage—a condition that may go undetected for years.

http://www.trans4mind.com/nutrition/pH.html

> **Comment:** Dr Otto Warburg has demonstrated that alkaline body tissue holds 20% more oxygen than acidic tissue (see next chapter on oxygen).

It has been demonstrated that an acidic, anaerobic (lacking oxygen) body environment encourages the breeding of fungi, molds, bacteria, and viruses. Tissues degrade, and disease thrives in an acidic environment. It is one of the causes for every known disease.

According to a book written by Robert R. Barefoot and Carl J. Reich, MD,

- Most kids have a pH of 7.5.
- Over 50% of adults have a pH of 6.5 or lower.
- Cancer patients usually have a pH of 4.5.

Here is a poll of 1,718 people with cancer who tested their saliva and provided their results.

http://www.alkalizeforhealth.net/salivaphtest.htm

Test Your Saliva pH. If you have cancer, what is your saliva pH? (1,718 votes total)

http://images.google.ca/imgres?imgurl=http://www.onlinecancerinfo.com/images/foodchart.jpg&imgrefurlhttp://www.onlinecancerinfo.com/docs/diet/pHbalance.htm&h=2353&w=3023&sz=1211&hl=en&start=16&usg=__pZhBuVX_IMGNBok_aDDjWOhvS2Q=&tbnid=teXAAlIbM9IVLM:&tbnh=117&tbnw=150&prev=/images%3Fq%3Dalkaline%2Bfood%2Bchart%26gbv%3D2%26hl%3Den%26sa%3DG

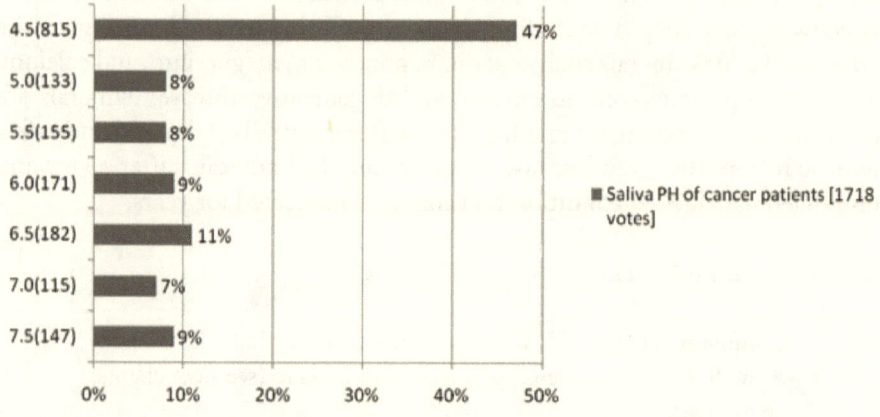

Saliva PH of cancer patients [1718 votes]

Subsequent research by Keith Brewer, PhD and H.E. Satori has shown that cancer cannot exist when the body's pH is raised to 8.0.

Dr Brewer developed a protocol to therapeutically raise pH with the element cesium in conjunction with potassium.

http://www.webring.com/hub?ring=naturalcuresthey

> **Comment:** Cesium, which makes the body alkaline, is another sub-chapter near the end of this book.

Health Problems Caused by Acidosis

If you have a health problem, it is possible that you are suffering from acidosis. Research shows that unless the body's pH level is slightly alkaline, the body cannot heal itself. So, no matter what means you choose to take care of your health, it will not be effective unless the pH level is balanced. If your body's pH is not balanced, for example, you cannot assimilate vitamins, minerals, and food supplements effectively. Your body pH affects everything.

Acidosis will decrease the body's ability to absorb minerals and other nutrients, slow the transportation of oxygen, decrease the energy production in the cells, decrease its ability to repair damaged cells, decrease its ability to detoxify heavy metals, make tumor cells thrive, and make it more susceptible to fatigue and illness.

An acidic pH can occur from an acid-forming diet, emotional stress, toxic overload, and/or immune reactions, or any process that deprives the cells of oxygen and other nutrients. The body will try to compensate for acidic pH by using alkaline minerals. If the diet does not contain enough minerals to compensate, a buildup of acids in the cells will occur. Acidosis can cause such problems as:

slower digestion and elimination
yeast/fungal overgrowth (see chapter on understanding *Candida*)
lack of energy and fatigue
lower body temperature
tendency to get infection
loss of drive, joy and enthusiasm
depressive tendencies
easily stressed
pale complexion
headaches, inflammation of the corneas and eyelids, loose and painful teeth
inflamed, sensitive gums
mouth and stomach ulcers
cracks at the corners of the lips
excess stomach acid
gastritis
nails are thin and splitting
dull looking hair with split ends and is falling out
dry skin or skin that is easily irritated
leg cramps and spasms

cardiovascular damage
weight gain, obesity, and diabetes
bladder conditions, kidney stones
immune deficiency
acceleration of free radical damage
hormonal problems
premature aging
osteoporosis and joint pain
aching muscles and lactic acid buildup
low energy and chronic fatigue

http://www.trans4mind.com/nutrition/pH.html

> **Comment:** Acidosis causes a list of problems because it affects every part of the body.

For example, osteoporosis is very confusing for many people. Most people think they can eliminate it by increasing their consumption of milk and dairy products. However, in the countries where the consumption of dairy products is very low, the prevalence of osteoporosis is very rare. Osteoporosis is in fact an acidosis problem. As the body becomes more acidic, to protect against the event of heart attack, stroke, illness, or even cancer, the body attempts to remain healthy. So, it steals calcium from the bones, teeth, and tissue. As bone mass becomes depleted, this is what we call osteoporosis. As we saturate the body with calcium, this brings the alkaline pH up and drops the acid levels down.

http://www.thewolfeclinic.com/phbalancearticle.html

> **Comment:** Food poisoning or botulism causes flurosynthesis. This is what happens when all of the bacteria in your body goes haywire. The end result is a highly acidic (and low oxygen) body.

> **Comment on the Lactic Acid Burning Sensation:** Lack of oxygen causes the body to steal it from the cells. This causes the cells to become acidic very quickly as the cells go from 7.1 to 6.5 pH, stimulating free nerve endings and giving the sensation of pain. The only way to reverse the sensation is to stop the work being drawn on the muscles or a rapid and continuous supply of oxygen to the muscles. Therefore, we know that acidity causes lack of oxygen, and lack of oxygen causes acidity.

http://www.healthynewage.com/balance-your-ph.htm

Why Acid-Alkaline Body Balance Is a Must

To stay healthy for life, your body needs to be in an acid-alkaline balance state. Cancer cannot survive in an acid-alkaline balance state. Restored to its proper alkaline state, the body takes care of business all by itself. A combination of detoxification (see chapter on detoxification), fresh raw foods, and exercise is the foundation for healing. Oxygen is routinely used in laboratories to kill off cancerous and viral cell cultures. Dr. Otto Warburg from Germany has demonstrated that low levels of oxygen in the cells cause cancer, and that unlike healthy cells that use oxygen for energy, cancer cells use fermentation to create energy. And thus, cancer cells thrive in an acidic environment.

www.NewHealthFrontier.com

Steps You Can Immediately Take to Improve Your pH

Fortunately, it is pretty easy to immediately change your pH for the better and make it more alkaline. The first step is to understand which of the foods you are eating and the drinks you are drinking are acidic and which are alkaline. Then it is simply a matter of eliminating some of the more acidic foods you are eating and adding in more alkaline foods.

In addition to decreasing the amount of acid foods you eat and increasing the amount of alkaline foods you eat, one of the best ways to immediately begin changing your pH is to drink *"green drinks"*. You can make these by simply adding a powder that is made up of a whole host of vegetables that are highly alkaline to a glass of water.

http://ezinearticles.com/?How-Body-pH-Can-Affect-Your-Energy-Levels&id=4670

The current typical Western diet is largely composed of acid-forming foods (proteins, cereals, sugars). Alkaline-producing foods such as vegetables are eaten in much smaller quantities. Stimulants like tobacco, coffee, tea, and alcohol are also extremely acidifying. Stress and physical activity (either insufficient or excessive amounts) also cause acidification.

Many foods are alkaline-producing by nature, but manufactured processed foods are mostly acid-producing. It is important to consume at least 60% alkaline-producing foods in our diet in order to maintain good health. We need plenty of fresh fruits and particularly vegetables (alkaline-producing) to balance our necessary protein intake (acid-producing). And we need to avoid processed, sugary, or simple-carbohydrate foods, not only because they are acid-producing but also because they raise blood sugar levels too quickly (high glycemic index therefore fattening); plus they tend to be nutrient-lacking and may be toxic as well.

http://www.trans4mind.com/nutrition/pH.html

> **Comment:** Aside from making urine, our kidneys control blood pressure, the amount of water, and the chemical balance of the blood. Therefore, our kidneys assist in controlling the acidity or pH balance of our blood. When the blood is too acidic, our kidneys make bicarbonate to restore the blood's pH balance, which it then excretes into the urine. On top of the kidney, adrenal glands control many things such as sugar and fat metabolism with hormones such as estrogen, progesterone, steroids, cortisol, cortisone, and chemicals such as adrenalin (*epinephrine*) and norepinephrine.
>
> So if I know that my diet is very acidic, and working backward, I have to assume that I have caused a tremendous amount of stress to my kidney in at least two ways: (i) by asking it to filter too much junk/poisons; and (ii) by having a poor pH balance (associated with bad diet and stress). This caused a constant supply of bicarbonate to be required (and made) while my body attempted to reverse this condition. In the end, an acidic body caused a tremendous amount of stress to my kidneys.
>
> My suggestions are to find a food pH balance chart. Pick the foods that you like on the alkaline side, and start eating more of them. You will probably also notice some of your favorite foods are very acidic. It seems redundant to say you should eat less of them. Second, read Kevin Trudeau's *"Natural Cures they Don't Want You to Know About"*. It is all about diet and detoxifying, which is a large part of pH balance. Third, consider purchasing a water ionizer (see chapter on ionized water a.k.a. alkaline water). If your goal is to deal with cancer or just be healthy, I suggest that you make yourself more aware of your diet and your pH level. If you do not, you just might destroy a kidney before you turn thirty.
>
> **Comment:** At the end of this book, you will find a food pH chart. It is only to be used a rough guide as I suspect its accuracy is lacking due to conflicting information, which may be related to the multitude of testing variables.

CHAPTER 9

Why Oxygenation is Important

Comment: Oxygen is like having "central air in your house" or opening a window. You need to let some fresh air in, or else the whole house becomes stagnant. A lack of oxygen creates the perfect environment for bacteria, molds and viruses to thrive. Dr. Otto Warburg has also demonstrated that a body lacking in oxygen is the perfect environment for cancer to thrive in. Oxygen is also a major detoxifier. Your body can only live for about four minutes without it. Your brain can live maybe eight minutes. A lack of oxygen is also the reason for migraine headaches.

By mass, human cells consist of 65 to 90% water (H_2O), and a significant portion is composed of carbon-containing organic molecules. Oxygen therefore contributes a majority of a human body's mass, followed by carbon. Ninety-nine percent of the mass of the human body is made up of the six elements: oxygen (65%), carbon (18%), hydrogen (10%), nitrogen (3%), calcium (1.5%), and phosphorus (1.2%).

http://en.wikipedia.org/wiki/Abundance_of_the_chemical_elements

Comment: Oxygen has two weak shells with eight "*neutrally charged*" electrons. This is the reason oxygen "*bonds*" so easily to itself and other things.

Your muscles need oxygen so badly; if they do not get enough during exercise, they will take it from hemoglobin in the working muscle. This lowers pH in the body and also causes lactic acid, which you then have to get out of your system as well. It also triggers positive hormonal changes, which could explain why exercising regularly keeps us young.

Oxygenation: The presumption is that human disease, including cancer (which represents 33% of deaths), is caused by a deficit of tissue oxygen (which, as we spoke about before, can be caused by acidosis). According to proponents, hypoxia results in anaerobic fermentation, a loss of capacity for oxidative detoxification of toxins and metabolic products and failure of the immune system in killing off invading bacteria and viruses.

http://www.quackwatch.org/01QuackeryRelatedTopics/Cancer/oxygen.html

> **Comment:** Smoking causes 33% of cancer patients (lack of oxygen) through dehydration/ oxification and toxic input directly from smoke. It is important to point out as well that many people do not breathe properly. Most people breathe into their chests, when what they should be doing, is breathing into their stomachs.

All of us, to some degree and at some time, suffer the effects of low energy. Plus, most know that oxygen levels where we live and work are often less than optimal.

And just going outside is not the answer either, for unless you live in pristine wilderness, oxygen concentrations have been measured as much as 30% below normal in and around major cities. This means with each breath, we take in less oxygen but most actually need a lot more.

As if this was not bad enough, most people have poor breathing habits. Most commonly, a failure to breathe effortlessly and with the entire diaphragm and lung, which further reduces the volume of air and oxygen we take in. The result, oxygen deficiency exerts an incalculable effect on our health and overall performance.

Oxygen also stimulates the growth and beneficial effects of friendly bacteria our bodies' need to maintain good health.

Oxygen decreases the growth and negative effects of pathogenic (harmful) invaders. Nearly all known pathogenic bacteria and viruses are unable to survive in an oxygen-rich environment.

http://www.breathing.com/e3live.htm

Oxygen includes 21% of the atmosphere at all altitudes. The remaining atmosphere consists of 78% nitrogen and 1% traces of other gases. Oxygen under normal conditions is an odorless, colorless, tasteless, noncombustible gas. It is the single most important element of our planet.

At each breath, we fill our lungs with air. Millions of tiny sacs (known as 'alveoli') in our lungs inflate like tiny balloons. In the minutely thin walls enclosing each sac are microscopic capillaries through which blood is constantly transported from the lungs to every cell in the body. The blood carries the oxygen extracted from the air in the lungs to every part of the body. Because the body has no way to store oxygen, it leads to breath-to-breath existence.

The human body must have oxygen to convert fuel (the carbohydrates, fats, and proteins in our diet) into heat, energy, and life. The conversion of body fuels into life is similar to the process of combustion; fuel and oxygen is consumed while heat and energy are generated. This process is known as metabolism.

The rate of metabolism, which determines the need for and consumption of oxygen, depends on the degree of physical activity or mental stress on the individual. Not all people require the same amount of oxygen. A man walking at a brisk pace will consume about four times as much oxygen as he will while sitting quietly. Under severe exertion or stress, he could possibly be consuming eight-fold more oxygen as he would when resting.

Acidity and low oxygen are requirements for good fermentation. They are also requirements for cancer to grow and flourish. Without them, cancer will die. When cells do not get enough of the oxygen they need to create energy, they ferment blood sugar for energy instead. But when that blood sugar breaks down into lactic acid, it raises the acidity, the pH level of your body.

Gilles Coulombe, Published: 4/19/2008

http://www.buzzle.com/articles/acid-alkaline-balance-is-a-must.html

Why Do Our Bodies Actually Need Oxygen?

In the cells of our body are lots of organelles (cell organs). One of these is called "*mitochondria*". They are in every cell and are known as the powerhouses of the cell. Mitochondria take different elements and nutrients from the cell (the cell gets them from your blood and your blood gets them from your food, which is why we eat) and send them through a mitochondrial factory. This "assembly line" is called the Krebs cycle. At the end of this assembly line, you can find the most basic source of (animal) energy, called ATP (adenosine triphosphate).

So here we are, with a bunch of ATP. Now what? Well, you need to burn it and get all the energy out of it! In order to do that, guess what we need (this is where you scream "OXYGEN!"). Yep, just like burning a piece of wood, any type of burning requires oxygen. So we breathe. We make a lot of ATP, so we need to inhale a lot of oxygen to get the energy from our little ATP's.

http://www.snyderhealth.com/oxygen.htm

> **Comment:** A lack of oxygen can cause migraine headaches. This also relates to cancer because with a lack of oxygen, you facilitate the perfect environment for cancer to thrive in. First, let's consider the effects of high-altitude or mountain sickness (which we know unquestionably is caused by a drop in oxygen pressure).

Sometimes people get sick at high altitudes, such as in the mountains. This is called mountain sickness or high-altitude sickness.

What are the symptoms?

Symptoms usually begin within forty-eight hours of arriving at high altitude, the higher the altitude, the greater the effects. People can notice effects when they go to an altitude of seven to eight thousand feet. If you have heart disease (such as heart failure) or lung disease (such as emphysema), you may experience the symptoms at lower altitudes. Symptoms include *headaches*, breathlessness, fatigue, lack of oxygen, nausea or vomiting, imbalance in pH, inability to sleep, hormone imbalance, and edema (swelling of the face, hands and feet).

Both heart rate and breathing rate increase as the body tries to send more oxygen to its tissues. At very high altitudes, body fluid can leak into the brain (called brain or cerebral edema) or into the lungs (pulmonary edema). Both these conditions can be serious or even life-threatening.

http://www.americanheart.org/presenter.jhtml?identifier=4618

Altitude sickness is caused by reduced partial pressure of oxygen. The percentage of oxygen in air remains essentially constant with altitude at 21% but the air pressure (and therefore the number of oxygen molecules) drops with altitude. Altitude sickness usually does not affect persons traveling by air because modern aircraft passenger compartments are pressurized.

http://en.wikipedia.org/wiki/Altitude_sickness

Comment: Many people suggest that migraines are caused by lack of oxygen. It is my experience that this is related to an acidic body that cannot hold or distribute oxygen (or a lack of vitamin B12 and magnesium, according to the "latest" research). Consider this: Alcohol and most food we eat create an acidic environment, which lowers oxygen content and absorption rate in the body. This is why pills do not work effectively in this environment (at best, they might trick you pain receptors). Consequently, we experience nausea and possibly throw up every time we suffer a migraine. This explains why people with migraines want to stop moving or sit down (as more oxygen is required for activity than rest). Consider this as well: People who predominantly get migraines are sensitive to weather; i.e., rain coming, or a drop in barometric pressure, or a drop in oxygen pressure! Another thing that occurs when it is dry in the winter, your lungs have a more difficult time getting oxygen. This may explain why hot showers that increase the ambient humidity allow your lungs to absorb more oxygen, thereby providing a positive and immediate response on your migraines. It is because your can breathe better. This suggests that migraines are contributed to by a lack of oxygen.

Comment: The primary function of vitamin B12 is to produce red blood cells (which carry oxygen) and is also a nitric oxide scavenger (which causes vasodilatation or the expansion of blood vessel walls). A lack of B12 will cause anemia, which is a condition that occurs when you have an abnormally low amount of red blood cells. Anemia makes it difficult for your blood to carry oxygen. Migraines are caused by a lack of oxygen (moreover, your body's ability to carry and transport it).

Comment on Magnesium: Magnesium in adults is comprised of 0.05% of its body weight. Low magnesium is found in the brain tissue of individuals who suffer from migraine headaches. Magnesium helps to maintain tone in the blood vessels. Magnesium is a natural relaxant to both muscle and nerve cells (relaxed muscles allow for better blood flow and thus, oxygen transportation) while also being a "bronchodilator" (it relaxes and opens the bronchial track for easier breathing).

In one particular study, 50% of participants with an acute migraine headache attack had low magnesium levels in plasma.[1] Another comparative study concerning women who suffered from menstrual migraine headache attacks, used magnesium supplementation to provide an effective reduction in pain caused from migraine attacks.[2] Intravenous magnesium is of great benefit for treating acute migraine headache attacks, and, in some cases, will cause instant relief from symptoms.

1. Mauskop A and Altera BM. Role of magnesium in pathogenesis and treatment of migraine. Clin Neuro Sci. 1998; 5(1): 24-27.
2. Facchinetti F et al. Magnesium prophylaxis of menstrual migraine: effects on intracellular magnesium. Headache 1991 May; 31(5): 298-301.

> **Comment:** So magnesium is directly related to blood flow and indirectly related to oxygen transportation.

> **Comment:** Magnesium is vital for *"oxidative phosphorylation."* According to Wikipedia, oxidative phosphorylation is a metabolic pathway that uses energy released by the oxidation of nutrients to produce adenosine triphosphate (ATP). Although the many forms of life on earth use a range of different nutrients, almost all carry out oxidative phosphorylation to produce ATP, the molecule that supplies energy for metabolism. To put it simply, magnesium is vital to the process that uses oxygen to burn vitamins and produce ATP ("energy").

http://en.wikipedia.org/wiki/Oxidative_phosphorylation

Consider some of the deficiencies to illustrate further the relationship between magnesium and oxygen. Symptoms of magnesium deficiency:

sensitivity to sound
muscular twitching
rapid heart rate
aching muscle
muscle weakness
convulsion
depression

grouchiness
vomiting
insomnia
irritability
hyperacidity
anxiety
confusion
disorientation
hypertension

http://hubpages.com/hub/Function of Magnesium in the Body

> **Comment:** The symptoms for altitude sickness (which we know are caused by a lack of oxygen) seem to run in parallel to the symptoms for B12 and magnesium deficiency, which seem to run parallel to the symptoms of migraine headaches. Therefore, I suggest that migraines are caused by a lack of oxygen.

Tension headaches are very common and are most likely in adults and adolescents. A tension headache is where there is muscle tightness in certain areas in the head, scalp, or neck accompanied by pain or discomfort in the same place. The symptoms are a dull, all-over pain, which often feels like a tight band or vice on the head. Such headaches are caused by the tension in the neck and scalp muscles and may be as a result of stress, depression, head injury, or anxiety. They can even be caused by the head being held in the same position for too long such as when typing or using a computer, doing fine work with the hands, or using a microscope. Even going to bed in too cold a room or sleeping with the neck in an abnormal position may bring on this tension headache.

There are several other causes such as:

eye strain
tiredness
alcohol and/or heavy smoking
too much caffeine
sinus infection or nasal congestion
colds and flu
insuffient rest
poor posture
anxiety

fatigue
hunger
overexertion

http://www.medicalnewstoday.com/articles/73936.php

http://www.medicinenet.com/tension_headache/article.htm#tocc

Comment on Tension Headaches: I used to be a regular migraine sufferer. Along with my migraines, I almost always had stiffness in my neck and back, i.e., knots caused from tension, obstructing the transportation of oxygen, specifically to my head. The major symptoms of "tension headaches" again also appear to be contributed to by lack of oxygen. A cold room causes headaches by constricting muscles, which may hold less oxygen as well as transport blood (and oxygen) more slowly. Tiredness causes poor posture, which causes us to yawn because our bodies are craving oxygen. Menstrual cramps and headaches also may be contributed to by a lack of blood, which as we know is the carrier of oxygen. Alcohol causes acidity, which we know decreases your body's ability to hold oxygen. Sinus infection or nasal congestion makes it harder to breathe oxygen. Anxiety causes muscle tightness, which uses up oxygen and also slows the transportation of oxygen. It seems to me that one of the underlying "causes" for tension and migraine headaches are basically the same, namely, a lack or limitation of adequate oxygen to the brain.

Comment: Seeing as how we are talking about tension headaches, we might as well talk a little bit about massage therapy. Stress and specifically knots make it difficult for your body to expel poisons, (never mind the distribution of oxygen, vitamins and minerals). Any form of stress or tension increases free radical production because muscles contract and require more oxygen. "You can prevent cancer." Michael Colgan PhD. (Adapted from materials provided by Blackwell Publishing)

We can establish this trend when we go to the massage therapist and are told that we "should breathe deeply while receiving the massage". If you have ever experienced this, you will agree that that increased breathing has a dramatic effect on the speed at which the knots dissipate, suggesting again that a lack of oxygen is an underlying cause of tension headaches.

Oxygen Therapy for Migraine Headaches

Two types of oxygen therapy may offer relief to people who suffer from disabling migraine and cluster headaches.

A review of a number of studies evaluated normobaric oxygen therapy and hyperbaric oxygen therapy in the treatment of migraines and cluster headaches. Normobaric therapy consists of patients inhaling pure oxygen at normal room pressure, and hyperbaric therapy involves patients breathing oxygen at higher pressure in a specially designed chamber.

Three studies reported a significant increase in the proportion of patients who had relief with hyperbaric oxygen compared to sham therapy. For cluster headaches, two studies found that a significantly greater proportion of patients had relief of their headaches after fifteen minutes of normobaric therapy compared to sham therapy.

About 6 to 7% of men and 15 to 18% of women suffer from severe migraine headaches, and cluster headaches affect about 0.2% of the population.

Science Blog July 16, 2008, Cochrane Database of Systematic Reviews July 16, 2008, Issue 3 (George H. Sands, MD. Beth Israel Medical Center New York, New York)

Dr. Kudrow investigated patients with cluster headaches and found that of them, forty-two outpatients were treated with 100% oxygen at a flow of seven liters per minute. Seventy-five percent of these patients had complete or almost complete cessation of head pain within fifteen minutes for at least seven of ten attacks.

Oxygen treatment of headaches was first mentioned in literature in 1939. Mr. Charles E. Rhein, Linde Air Products Co., reported to Dr. Alvarez at the Mayo Clinic in Rochester, MN the successful treatment of severe "migraine" attacks by breathing pure oxygen. Subsequently, Dr. Alvarez noted that the treatment with 100% oxygen at a flow of six to eight liters a minute would often produce relief. Sometimes patients would not be able to obtain relief with this treatment, whereas at other times, they would. In 1940, Dr. Alvarez reported the treatment of over one hundred persons suffering from headache attacks. They were treated with oxygen with a nasal type of mask and a flow of six to eight liters a minute. He found that 80% of "migraine" headaches were completely or significantly attenuated.

http://www.airheads1.com/Headaches.html

> **Comment:** I suggest the reason for less than 100% efficacy with oxygen therapy has to do with either a difficulty in the absorption or a limited distribution of oxygen.

> **Comment:** I asked my acupuncture doctor what the cause of grinding teeth was. His response was stress and/or lack of oxygen. I find a strange correlation between this and memories of two friends of mine who used to grind their teeth. Both of these friends used to grind their teeth only after long nights of drinking. The reason that I mention this is because both of these people used to drink beer, which is very acidic (pH 2.5). As I have said earlier, a high acid content will cause a deficiency of oxygen in the body (see chapter on pH). Interestingly, I spoke to one of those friends about six months ago, and he told me that he just had a cancerous tumor removed. Fortunately, he is doing very well and is still very happy.

> **Comment:** Try this: Slowly take in ten DEEP breaths. You felt a tingle in your body, didn't you? This is increased oxygen in your body allowing for better electrical impulse transmission. Remember that bioelectric thing? That is a good thing.

> **Comment:** Having done so much reading on oxygen for migraines, it seemed like a good time to test it out for myself. I found out very quickly that most companies who sell oxygen machines require a prescription? A prescription to breathe oxygen? Having already complained for years about migraines, I thought it would be no problem to go to my doctor and get this prescription. Well, my family doctor told me that she had never prescribed an oxygen machine to anyone before and did not know anything about the subject. I would need to see a neurologist to get more information (who I expected would have similar information as my family doctor and try to prescribe what they know already, such as pain-blockers known as drugs with side-effects).

Oxygen As A Drug

The FDA classifies oxygen as a drug. Therefore, both its application and the devices used to administer it fall under the FDA's jurisdiction. As a drug, oxygen can be administered only on the order of a physician.

http://www.netnet.net/mums/HBOregs.htm

> **Comment:** After three months of computer time and many phone calls, I finally find out that over 95% oxygen is classified as a drug. Machines that produce less than 95% oxygen do not qualify as a drug. Why did this take me months of research? Why did my family doctor not know this about oxygen? Why is this information not more readily available?

Nobel Prize winner Otto Warburg led us to the knowledge that *cancer lives in a low oxygen environment* like most bacteria. Every time Otto Warburg lowered the oxygen level by 35% in a healthy cell, it became cancerous. Based on his work, he proposed the use of vitamin E as a possible curb to the incidence of cancer, since vitamin E reduces the cells' need for oxygen. It is a good point, but why not increase the oxygen levels in a healthy cell? For example, one could use germanium organic 132, a trace element that increases the amount of oxygen in a cell. He found that the presence of increased amounts of oxygen inhibits the spread of cancer cells and eventually cause them to die.

http://www.stopcancer.com/cancer&ph1a.htm#UNDERSTANDING%20 THE%20BASIC%20PROBLEMS%20OF%20CANCER%20AND%20 ILLINESS

Based on the research and findings to date, our view of the essence of germanium is as follows:

It provides free electrons as a mother antioxidant. It neutralizes positive charges, mops them up, and discharges them in conjunction with converting cellular and tissue toxins to water. It should be noted that toxins arise from consuming any food, since some of our food remains as *unburnt cellular debris*' the germanium completes this 'burning process' by donating electrons and conserving cellular oxygen. These processes are so fundamental to the preservation and restoration of health that this 'electronic' therapy is one of the most potent available in a single remedy for many diseases and health maintenance.

Germanium enhances immunity and is a prime anti-aging remedy. It also greatly enriches oxygen in the living body.

http://www.regenerativenutrition.com/content.asp?id=441

Comment: If you want to avoid a migraine, try lowering your acid intake, increasing your vitamin intake, and drinking more water (which contains oxygen). This will allow you to absorb and move oxygen around your body more effectively. The other thing you might do to get more oxygen is purchase an oxygen machine. I recommend that you stay away machines that require refill (and explosive) oxygen tanks. Get yourself an oxygen "concentrator" instead.

Comment on Coenzyme Q10, CoQ10, Ubiquinone, Vitamin Q: Assisting with the production of ATP, CoQ10 is a major source of energy for the cells. It also acts as an antioxidant that enhances the immune system. CoQ10 also facilitates the release of oxygen and is used for anti-aging. This may explain why it can be used as a preventative to fight migraine headaches as well as cancer.

Comment: If you need to fight cancer, you need to consider your oxygen. A large portion of your body consists of it. Remember, cancer cannot survive in a high oxygen environment. Its weak outer shell gives it the ability to bond easily with other molecules. This means it works in almost the same way as antioxidants, but instead of giving up an electron, oxygen will "share" its electrons with other molecules, thereby, giving oxygen the ability to convert free radicals into a more stable form. Also, we have learned that oxygen is a major detoxifier and represents a large part of the cycle that converts ATP into cellular energy. Migraine headaches are just one sign that your body is being deprived of the oxygen that it requires. Needless to say, if you are going to deal with cancer, you had better make sure that your body is getting plenty of oxygen.

CHAPTER 10

Understanding Candida (Candidiasis)

Comment: Candida is like mold in your house. Reduce the oxygen, adjust the temperature (pH), fire the butler (immune system), termites eat holes (free radicals) and mold has the perfect environment to thrive. If your body is in a state where an overgrowth of bad bacteria can thrive, then it is also in a state where cancer can thrive. If you are going to fight cancer, there is a high probability that you will need to fight a Candida infection first.

Comment: Candida is another rarely discussed problem with severe ramifications. The effects and the cause (antibiotics and an acidic diet) are not widely considered in Western medicine, but is considered a major topic of discussion to those outside. If 60% of the population is eating a poor diet and is obese, then no doubt many of us have lost control of this at some point. Candida is an overgrowth of bad bacteria, amplified by an acidic diet and/or antibiotics (Just like the ones I was prescribed for my prostate infection).

Many medical conditions in our modern world can compromise our immune systems: excessive use of antibiotics or steroids (like prednisone), high sugar diets, diabetes, oral contraceptives, overly acidic pH levels from poor diet and stress, hormone imbalances, and exposure to environmental toxins (often molds). Our exposure to all these modern traps sets our bodies up for the fall into this fungal yeast overgrowth.

When our immune systems are compromised, the normal yeast present in our bodies, called *Candida*, can "morph" from being a beneficial yeast into a harmful fungus. This fungal yeast can quickly grow out of the balance that nature intended and overwhelm the beneficial flora (acidophilus—type friendly bacteria) that normally keeps natural yeast levels in check.

This new fungal form of yeast develops rhizoids (long burrowing legs) that hook into and can even penetrate the mucus membranes in the intestinal tract and cause serious bowel damage and pain. They can also enter the bloodstream and cause serious infection of vital organs.

As time goes on, the morphed fungal yeast may burrow right through the intestinal wall. This condition, called leaky gut syndrome, allows partially digested proteins and the yeast itself to travel into the bloodstream where they become toxins.

As undigested foods directly enter the bloodstream, this may further cause an immediate allergic reaction to certain foods. Once the yeast infection has access to the whole body, you have systemic Candida or systemic candidiasis.

> **Comment:** After I was told I had a prostate infection, I was given a month's supply of heavy antibiotics. Shortly after that, I felt like my body was starting to turn to stone. I could not think straight. Just about every part of my body ached. This, I believe, was a severe Candida infection that did not go away until I changed my diet drastically and started a daily regime of probiotics (good bacteria). Some of the symptoms of a Candida overgrowth (most of which I experienced) are:

constant fatigue/brain "fog" that easily overwhelms mental tasks (cognitive impairment)
anxiety
rectal itching
hyperactivity
earaches
muscle weakness
oral thrush (a white film on tongue or in the mouth)
abdominal pain (intestinal Candida)
bloating and indigestion
constant craving for something sweet
joint pain with arthritis-like symptoms chronic sinus drainage
weight loss or gain and the inability to change it
acid reflux/indigestion
fungi on the finger—or toe-nails
urinary infections
itching red eyes

Candida skin rashes on the body (eczema, atopic dermatitis)
Candida rash inside the ears or around the groin area
anal or vaginal itching
hair loss and vision problems
depression and mood swings

http://www.candidasupport.org/?gclid=CLfkqeaf5JQCFQbJsgodTzN6Rg

> **Comment:** There is no doubt to me that Candida overgrowth
> was a major reason for the problems that occurred after receiving
> antibiotics for my prostate infection. Poor diet and two years of
> Percocets could not have helped much either.

The major waste product of Candida is *acetaldehyde*, which produces
ethanol. Ethanol may be great in cars, but in your body it causes excessive
fatigue, and reduces strength and stamina. In addition, it destroys enzymes
needed for cell energy and causes the release of free radicals that can damage
DNA.

Ethanol also inhibits the absorption of iron. Because iron is one of the most
important oxygen supports in the blood, ethanol in your body creates low oxygen
levels. And you know what happens when your body can not oxygenate well. It
seems that a Candida infection might be an important precursor for cancer.

http://www.cancerfightingstrategies.com/fungalconnection.html

The brain is the organ that is most frequently affected by Candida
symptoms, but it also has profound negative effects on these systems:

digestive
neurological
cardiovascular
respiratory
reproductive
urinary
endocrine
lymphatic
musculoskeletal

Candida symptoms can vary from one person to another and often move
back and forth between systems within the same individual. One day, you may

experience symptoms in the musculoskeletal system; and the next day, it could be in your digestive system, and so on and so on.

A simple and effective and affordable way to test for Candida is called the "*spit test*." Here is how you can do it: As soon as you wake up in the morning, before you put anything in your mouth, get a glass of water in a clear glass that you can see through. Do not use chlorinated tap water. Collect saliva in your mouth with your tongue and spit it into the glass. Now keep an eye on your saliva in the glass for the next fifteen minutes, and observe what it does. If you see any of the following, then you have yeast colonies:

Your saliva stays at the top, and you see thin strands that look like strings or spider legs extending downward.

Your saliva sinks to the bottom and looks cloudy.

Your saliva is suspended midglass and looks like little specks are floating.

See the picture below for guidance.

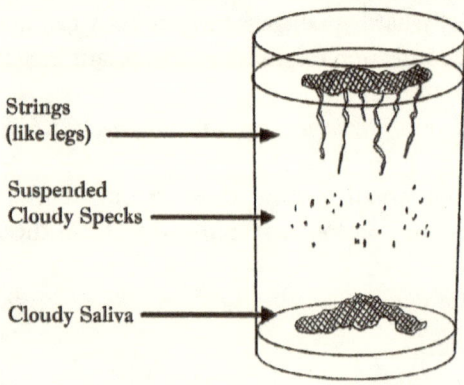

Strings (like legs)

Suspended Cloudy Specks

Cloudy Saliva

Candida is an insidious tricky yeast. Once you have an overgrowth, it can be extremely difficult to get under control. It takes patience, education and persistence.

http://www.holistichelp.net/candida.html

Some doctors implicate fungi as a cause of leukemia. In 1999, Meinolf Karthaus, MD, watched three different children with leukemia suddenly go into remission upon receiving a triple antifungal drug cocktail for their "secondary" fungal infections.

In 1997, Mark Bielski stated that leukemia, whether acute or chronic, is intimately associated with the yeast, Candida albicans, which mutates into a fungal form when it overgrows.

Doug Kaufmann asserts that fungi in foods may play a role in cancer. He has seen children become free of their documented leukemia once the child's parents simply changed the child's diet. Kaufmann's diet is based on the widely published problem of mycotoxin contamination of our grain foods. Kaufmann suggested that *antibiotics* may play a role in this. Antibiotics destroy the normal protective gut bacteria, allowing intestinal yeast and fungi to grow unchecked, resulting in Candida overgrowth. This can lead to immune suppression, symptoms of autoimmune diseases, or even cancer.

http://www.cancerfightingstrategies.com/fungalconnection.html

> **Comment:** One effective way to fight Candida bacteria is with probiotics (not antibiotics) that are strains of good bacteria required by your stomach and intestines. These probiotics should be taken before bed (when you are resting and not digesting), preferably on an empty stomach so that some of the bacteria have a chance to make their way into your intestines. Probiotics help with the digestion of foods by balancing the microflora in the gut. As such, they can also be used to assist travelers with diarrhea. However, I suggest not purchasing a probiotic support that is stored in the same food in which it is meant to break down; for example, yogurts with "probiotics added". By the time it gets to your stomach, there will be no more live bacteria left. (Once again, it seems to be all about money and marketing.) Probiotics can also be used to repopulate the digestive tract after a course of antibiotics has upset this balance; research has shown probiotics can prevent almost half of the infections that are common after antibiotic use.

Probiotics Support, Immune System and Digestion

Another important digestive and immune system component is the probiotics or friendly organisms that live in our intestinal tract. Healthy individuals will literally have pounds of friendly bacteria and other microorganisms living in their guts. Not only do the probiotics complete the digestive process by producing many vitamins, breaking down food and killing pathogens, but they also play a major role in the immune system itself. Some nutritionists say that they are the main component of the immune system, comprising 70% of the total immune system.

On the other hand, antibiotics and many other medications including chemotherapy, chlorinated water, birth control pills, and more kill the probiotics. This potential lack of friendly organisms is a primary cause of Candida fungal overgrowth. Even if you have been eating yogurt or taking acidophilus, you most likely still do not have enough. Very few yogurts contain live bacteria, and even in those that do, the bacteria in yogurt do not colonize the intestinal tract.

In addition, most probiotic supplements fail to deliver many live organisms into the intestines for two reasons. First, many of them die while the product sits on the shelves. Refrigeration is used to slow down their metabolism and to keep them alive, but studies consistently show that a great many of the live bacteria die in the bottle.

Second, even more destructive is the stomach environment wherein the acidity kills the friendly bacteria. Studies show that not much makes its way to the intestines.

http://www.cancerfightingstrategies.com/enzymes.html

> **Comment:** Most Western doctors will not acknowledge Candida as an underlying culprit. Every one of my doctors had never heard of the word before I asked them about it. They will however acknowledge *cachexia*, which I believe to be the exact same thing. According to Western medicine, cachexia has no cure.

Definition of Cachexia

Cachexia: Physical wasting of muscle mass with loss of weight and caused by disease. Patients with advanced cancer, AIDS and some other major chronic progressive diseases may appear cachectic. Cachexia is a wasting syndrome that causes weakness and a loss of weight, fat, and muscle. Anorexia (lack of appetite) and cachexia often occur together. Cachexia can occur in people who are eating enough but who cannot absorb the nutrients. Cachexia is not the same as starvation. A healthy person's body can adjust to starvation by slowing down its use of nutrients, but in cachectic patients, the body fails to make this adjustment.

http://www.medterms.com/script/main/art.asp?articlekey=11065

> **Comment:** Without good bacteria in your stomach, you will have a hard time digesting food and subsequently vitamins, minerals and nutrients. This will also cause you to constantly feel full; and the Candida will steal some of the vitamins, minerals, and nutrients from your food for themselves.

Cachexia is one of the most devastating symptoms of cancer, up to 75% of cancer patients suffer from this condition. It robs patients of their energy, quality of life, enjoyment, and ultimately sense of independence. Most patients afflicted with cancer cachexia are those with cancers of the upper gastrointestinal tract. These include cancers of the esophagus, stomach and pancreas. One study noted that 85% of all patients with pancreatic cancer develop cachexia and lose a median of 14.2% of their pre cancer weight just by the time of diagnosis. Average survival for patients diagnosed with pancreatic cancer is only nine to twelve months.

http://www.oncolink.org/resources/article.cfm?c=3&s=38&ss=164&id=828

> **Comment:** Most doctors do not know how to relieve these "cachectic" symptoms. All they have to offer is the suggestion that you cut back of sugars, the same sugars that feed bad bacteria and cause Candida. What they don't tell you is that you would be better off shifting towards a more alkaline diet and taking probiotics every night before bed. As I have said before, a Candida overgrowth is like a five star hotel for cancer. The conditions for cancer growth do not get much better. Candida represents again only one piece of the equation, but if you plan on fighting cancer (or being healthy for that matter), you need to address the Candida issue. The best way that this can be done is with a proper alkaline diet and nightly probiotic support (of which I recommend switching strains now and then for variety).

CHAPTER 11

Why Your Lymphatic System is Crucial

Comment: Your lymphatic system is the "other half" of your immune system (which is part of the final battle against cancer). Most of us have about twice as much lymph fluid as blood. This represents about 27% of your body's fluid. If it is not working, then it really does not matter what your blood is doing. Your lymphatic system is like the drains that remove waste in your home, such as the sink, the toilet and the washing machine. If you were to plug up the drains, waste would back up very quickly inside your home. Unlike your bloodstream that uses your heart to pump blood around your body, your lymphatic system can only move lymph fluid around by muscle contraction. This may be one of the reasons why a twenty minute walk every day is very healthy for you. Consider for a moment, if you will, that bras are known to cause breast cancer, or that regular breast massage prevents breast cancer. Is it possible that this is due largely in part to movement (or lack thereof) of lymphatic fluid?

Your lymphatic system is the reason that breast cancer is so harmful. It is due to the production of immune cells, lymphocytes, monocytes, and antibody producing plasma cells. Your immune system produces and distributes interstitial fluid. This is the solvent that bathes and surrounds the body's cells. This interstitial fluid contains sugars, amino acids, hormones, coenzymes, salts, neurotransmitters, fatty acids, and some waste products from the cells. Now try to imagine what would happen if this interstitial fluid or "lymphatic system" were to get infected with *Candida*?

It is easy to see the correlation between allergies and lymph nodes when you know a little bit about the lymphatic system. When considering the reasons for swollen lymph nodes, the first consideration is whether these nodes are localized in area of the body or generalized throughout the body. Swollen lymph nodes that are localized tend to be responding to the part of the body that is filtered by these nodes. A scratch on your toe can cause swollen lymph nodes in the back of your knee or even your groin if the infection is severe enough. Any trauma to your fingers is filtered by nodes in your elbow and armpit. If generalized lymph nodes are the problem, this would suggest that the body is dealing with a whole body issue such as a drug or allergic reaction, a bacterial, fungal or viral infection, or an autoimmune disease (lupus or arthritis). This may explain the link between allergies and lymph nodes, an overactive thyroid, a metabolic disease, or a malignancy such as leukemia.

Allergies and lymph nodes are just two of the potential causes of swelling. We all have hundreds of lymph nodes scattered throughout our bodies, which represent a critical part of our immune system. This extensive network of lymph nodes works as a powerful, intelligent filtration system to keep the inside of our bodies clean and healthy. Tiny vessels called lymph vessels carry foreign particles, germs, and any unhealthy or malignant cells to the lymph nodes where they are trapped. As lymph nodes become active in their attempt to destroy unwelcome material, they become enlarged, making them the perfect indicator that you have an infection of some sort. Swollen lymph nodes are most often found in the armpit, neck, or groin. It should be noted however that your lymphatic "system" does extend throughout your entire body.

Anonymous

> **Comment on Tonsils:** They are part of your lymphatic system. Lymphocytes and macrophages in the tonsils provide protection against harmful substances and pathogens that may enter the body through the nose or mouth. So many people have had them removed for "unknown" or mysterious "infection" (or swelling). The tonsils are lymph nodes and, therefore, part of your lymphatic system, which your body needs to operate. In all probability, the swollen lymph nodes are not the problem. Your lymph nodes swell because they are active and fighting to resolve another problem. When and if that initial problem is solved, the swelling in your lymph nodes will go away.

Comment: Candida *was* the cause of the pain in my groin. The inguinal region: the nodes in this area receive lymph from the legs, the outer portion of the genitalia, and the lower abdominal wall. This was the reason it was exacerbated by heavy antibiotics (for a prostate infection) in February 2008. The reason it was not found was that none of the specialists with whom I spoke were aware of its existence. They had never heard of Candida. I supposed then that they would also have to acknowledge that it is caused predominantly by antibiotics that kill probiotics, the good bacteria.

The following diagram of the lymphatic system from the knee to the belly button looks exactly like the pain chart I would have drawn during my experience. This would explain why the platinum coils they implanted in my abdomen on Dec 17, 2007, did little to relieve my pain. I never had varicose veins; the problem was a severe Candida infection from probably years of bad diet and the final dose of antibiotics for my prostate infection pushed me over the edge. I suggest that severe Candida was "jamming up" my lymphatic system, causing me to experience almost every physical pain imaginable.

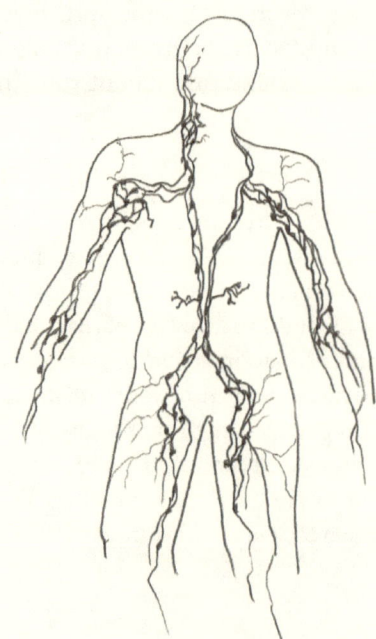

Immune System

Comment: Remember that the only way to move fluids around the lymphatic system is through "muscle contraction". Your lymphatic system is how you drain waste from your body and is complimentary to your immune system (which creates the waste). If you are going to deal with cancer, you need to keep the flow of toxins moving through your lymphatic system. Don't be a couch potato. You don't want that "junk" to sit there and facilitate the perfect environment for cancer or, worse yet, cause more cancer.

CHAPTER 12

Why Detoxification is Imperative

Comment: Detoxification is like having a garage sale. You pick up all the old, unwanted or unused items around your house to get rid of the clutter. It is another topic seldom addressed in Western medicine. Unquestionably, it was part of my recovery. If your colon, veins, arteries, and organs are blocked with junk, you will not absorb vitamins and minerals. As well, the "junk" will sit, then rot, and make you even sicker. This also applies to heavy metals in your body that cannot be removed without assistance. Heavy metals are especially bad because most, due to size, are able to cross the *"blood brain barrier".* This will cause an interruption in the signaling pathways that you require to think clearly and to operate your body (organs included). If you are going to deal with cancer, then you will need to address detoxification as well.

Nobel laureate Dr. Alexis Carrell of the Rockefeller Institute for Medical Research kept samples of heart tissue from a chicken embryo alive for twenty-nine years. The tissues were immersed in a medium solution from which they obtained all the necessary nutrients, and the cells excreted their metabolic wastes into the same solution. Each day, the old solution was discarded and replaced with fresh medium. After living for twenty-nine years, the chicken heart tissue died when the assistant forgot to change the polluted fluid. This is a powerful testimonial to the vital role and necessity of detoxification. Dr. Carrel concluded that "The cell is immortal. It is merely the fluid in which it floats that degenerates. Renew this fluid at regular intervals [detoxification], give the cell something on which to feed [proper diet and nutrition], and so far as we know, the pulsation of life may go on forever."

And indeed, a similar mechanism seems to apply in human cells. As they get nourished, they produce a certain amount of waste matter which, together with the toxins present in the ingested food, water, air, and other contaminants (chemical and radiation pollution) that we come in contact with, must be efficiently removed to prevent the body from slowly suffocating in its own refuse. "Detoxification is the final expulsion of waste materials through the various excretory organs. Detoxification takes place in the human body continually from birth throughout life. Life in the human body is maintained by the reproduction of cells, new cells arising to take the place of dead and worn-out ones. It is in a constant process of self-renewal. Cells are constantly being broken down, and cells are just as constantly being renewed or replaced." Toxins must be (and in a healthy state) eliminated continually and consistently both from the body and from our environment to allow genuine healing and health maintenance to take place.

Elnora van Winkle, a neurophysiologist, writes in her book *The Toxic Mind*, "Since the time of Hippocrates it has been understood that symptoms of most diseases, other than degenerative disorders where irreversible organic damage has been sustained, represent the efforts of the body to eliminate toxins. Any substance, endogenous or exogenous, that cannot be utilized by the cells is recognized as toxic and eliminated. When elimination is impaired, toxins accumulate. The cells adapt to toxicosis, but when levels of toxin become intolerable the body initiates a detoxification process. Toxicosis is the true disease, and what we call disease is remedial action, a complex of symptoms caused by the vicarious elimination of toxins. Recovery from disease is not because of remedies but in spite of them."

http://www.healingcancernaturally.com/detoxification.html

Types of Toxins in Your Body

There are several types of toxic buildups in the body that need to be dealt with when fighting cancer. First, there is cellular toxicity caused by the shunting of toxins into cells due to excess acidity in the blood and the inability to release toxins in the cells for that very same reason.

Next is heavy metal and chemical toxicity coming from years of exposure to highly toxic heavy metals and chemicals (like working in a glass factory). While many come from the environment, silver amalgam fillings, many vaccines, and some other drugs put mercury and other toxins into our body. For example, most large fish have elevated mercury levels. Elevated levels of heavy metals disrupt the immune system and *must* be dealt with when fighting cancer.

> **Comment:** After much effort, I acquired one of the top heavy metal cleansers. It was a combination of over seventy herbs and

vitamins that "attach" to metals so they are easier for the body to identify and push out. The first day of a thirty-day cleanse, I did a half dose to start. Hours later, I got a severe migraine and threw up most of the night. All I could taste was metal. It was like someone had melted a pop can down into liquid and put it in my mouth. It was quite the experience. Over the next few weeks of cleansing, I drank at least two liters of water and went to the sauna every day. By week two, I started to notice an orange discoloration on my sandals that would not wash off even with soap. By week four, my sandals looked like someone had spilt dark orange paint on them. There was no doubt that metals were being pushed out of my body. I also destroyed most of my white socks. In fact, I had to stop the cleanse on two occasions (I had done three months in total) because my lymphatic system got so jammed up it caused pain in some of my lymph nodes. The first time it was the lymph node in my left armpit. I had trouble breathing without pain for several days because it was so swollen. But, upon completing the cleansing, I noticed a very significant improvement in my ability to breathe and think, and my migraine headaches were attenuated.

There also was a toxic buildup in the colon of undigested foods and hardened fecal matter. Nutrient absorption was disrupted, and toxins sitting in that decaying mess were reabsorbed back into the body. This creates a constant stress on the immune system and a further load on the body's detoxification process. Colon cleaning needs to happen on the journey to good health.

http://www.cancerfightingstrategies.com/toxins.html

Comment: I also have completed two months of colon cleansing. This gave me the sweats and made me feel very bloated, but the positive effects afterwards were quite noticeable. There is no doubt to me that my food absorption has significantly improved since. Food also "moves" through my body much better (and faster) as well.

"Every tissue is fed by the bloodstream, which is supplied by the intestines. When the intestines are dirty, the blood is dirty, and so are the organs and tissues. It is the intestines that must be cared for first before any effective healing can take place."

Dr. Bernard Jensen

According to the FDA, the average American carries anywhere between five to twenty-two pounds of compacted fecal matter, (as foul toxic waste mucus) stuck in the folds of his/her colon (large intestine). This toxic mucus not only produces many free radicals (that can cause cells to mutate, which could lead to cancer), but also prevents our vital nutrients from being absorbed. Nature never intended for us to move those toxic substances through our system on a daily basis. Even the U.S. Department of Health and Human Services admits that 90% of Americans are walking around with clogged colons.

Almost ALL diseases are offered by this toxic cesspool in the colon. It is commonly known among medical circles that your colon is home base for almost every disease in the body. This stagnation is the reason that doctors recommend every adult over forty get a colonoscopy every year.

http://www.phwaterforhealth.com/sick.htm

> **Comment:** Many suggest that a clogged colon is the reason for prostate and colon cancer. Remember all that waste just sits there and rots. If colon cancer is your problem, then a colonoscopy is only going to confirm this fact, not relieve your body of the problem. One way to clean out your colon is a colonic. The other way is to remove the waste from your colon, using a colon cleanse. The one I did was to use a powder that expands in your colon and absorbs waste, along with a tea that you drink at night to help move things along. Don't even bother with any ingested cleanses that say they can do the job in three or seven days. It has taken many years to cause that waste to build up inside you, and there is no way you are going to clean it up in less than a month. For some people, it may take longer.

> **Comment:** As people start to get older, they get slower mentally. Why? What, in addition to general decay, would cause a slowing down of one's brainwave signals? Have you ever considered the causes of autism? Have you looked into mercury poisoning to its fullest? Are you aware that mercury (in the form of thimerosal, a mercury-based preservative) is in most, if not all, vaccines, albeit in minute amounts? There are many ways to detoxify the body. Oxygen, if you will recall, is a major detoxifier. There also are numerous cleanses that can be done in pill, powder and liquid form. In addition, you could drink ionized water (see chapter on ionized water) and/or go to the sauna

regularly. I also purchased a foot detox machine that pulls toxins out of the sweat glands in your feet. Whichever way, if you are going to fight cancer or just try to be healthy, you need to consider at least one, if not several, of these forms of detoxification. Detoxification is yet another major "piece" in the cancer equation.

CHAPTER 13

Water: The Major Component of Your Body

Comment: We are supposed to drink eight glasses or two liters of water a day. Few of us do, even thought it represents more than half of our body's mass. Water is essential to the functioning of every single cell and organ system in the human body. Water also is essential for the efficient elimination of waste products through the kidneys. Water can be considered like the humidity in your house. You need to have the right balance in order to be comfortable. Too little water and many of the body's functions will stop altogether. If you do somehow manage to drink too much (which is better than too little), you would lower salt concentration in the cells. The cells would swell, and you would still be out of balance. Water quality and intake represents a significant "piece" of the cancer equation.

Water and Dehydration

Total body water percentage decreases with age, resulting in inadequate cellular hydration. Most critical is the decrease in the ratio of intracellular hydration. The normal ratio is 60% intracellular, 40% extracellular. The reason for change in this ratio is due in part to an increase in fat along with a decrease in muscle and a decreased ability of the body to regulate sodium and water balance. With age, kidney function becomes less efficient in producing urine, and responses for conserving sodium weaken.

The body must continuously be in a proper state of hydration. Because 2.5 liters of water is lost each day through normal bodily functions, this must be replaced. There are two major issues that emphasize the need to keep the body adequately hydrated with water of the best quality, content, and structure so it can maintain homeostasis.

First, the water we put in our body must be able to prevent toxins and chemical substances from accumulating and creating destructive influences on cells. Water must bring all minerals and nutrients required for cell metabolism and remove any substances that can damage the cell. It must also be able to protect cell walls from damage and invasion.

Second, since water is involved in every function of the body, it must act as a conductor of electrochemical activity, such as neurotransmission, by moving water from one nerve cell to another smoothly and effectively.

Movement of water in the body between cells (extracellular fluid) is caused by *osmosis*. This is created by magnetic forces in the body, which keep the movement in balance. As water flows, changes in pressure create movement across the cell membranes. Any changes in pressure will allow proteins, minerals, and other nutrients being carried by the blood to escape into spaces between vessels and deprive the cells of their vital needs to sustain life. When water in the blood is contaminated with chemicals, it enters the cells and changes their structure, which, in turn, could lead to changes in DNA (pleomorphism). This is the start of the disease process, which is very similar to the aging process.

http://www.snyderhealth.com/water.htm

Percent of Water in the Body

100%	80%	70%	50%
Fetus	Baby at Birth	Normal Adult	Elderly Person

Comment: In the winter, my lips and hands were always very dry. I suggest the cause was not enough water. I used to use lip balm and hand cream all the time. However, I have now realized that if part of my body is dry, I need more water. Now that I am more aware of the situation, my lips and hands are rarely dry.

Our bodies use 2.5 liters of water at normal function in a mild climate. We should be drinking at least two liters of water a day. The most common signs of dehydration are headaches and fatigue. Our bodies prioritize when water is limited, so areas and organs low on the list just lose out.

Water is the only source of hydration. Not all liquids have a hydrating ability compared to water. For example, sodas, coffee, tea and alcohol actually will cause you to be more dehydrated. We need to drink more water. We need to drink better water.

http://www.phwaterforhealth.com/sick.htm

Comment: Ever since I bought a shower filter, it has reduced the amount of cleaning I need to do. I always thought that "scum" in the shower was from soap. Now, I realize it is from dirty city water. Consider the reason why so many car washes now have "streak-free" rinse water. They are now using a water filter (which also explains the decrease in water pressure). The car washes no longer leave streaks on your car. So, what is "*in*" the water that does?

The Environmental Working Group in 2005 tested the water in forty-two states. They detected 260 contaminants in the water supplies. Of those, 141 were unregulated chemicals for which public health officials have no safety standards, much less methods for removing them.

http://environment.about.com/od/healthenvironment/a/tap_water_safe.htm

Comment: A large part of your body is water. It is second in importance only after oxygen. It is essential to the functioning of every single cell and organ system in the human body (including your immune and lymphatic system). These are just a few of the reasons that you need to have the right intake of water to be healthy and/or win your fight with cancer. Without water, you would surely be dead in a week.

CHAPTER 14

Why Chlorine is Your Enemy

Comment: If you filled your humidifier with chlorine, everything near it would slowly deteriorate. Sadly, chlorine is being used to clean our water. It amazes me that there is any debate on whether or not chlorine is bad. Chlorine does not remove anything from the water, it simply breaks it down! You would certainly not ingest chlorine in large quantities because it does break things down. So, why is it okay in small quantities? Another part of good health and the cancer equation is the removal of chlorine from your diet.

"Long-term drinking of chlorinated water appears to increase a person's risk of developing bladder cancer as much as 80%," according to a study published in the *Journal of the National Cancer Institute*. Some forty-five thousand Americans are diagnosed every year with bladder cancer.

St. Paul Dispatch & Pioneer Press, December 17.

"The drinking of chlorinated water has finally been officially linked to an increased incidence of colon cancer. An epidemiologist at Oak Ridge Associated Universities completed a study of colon cancer victims and non-cancer patients and concluded that the drinking of chlorinated water for 15 years or more was conducive to a high rate of colon cancer."

Health Freedom News, January/February 1987

http://www.pure-earth.com/chlorine.html

"Cancer risks among people drinking chlorinated water is 93% higher than among those whose water does not contain chlorine."

Sainaw Hospital, Dr. JM Price, MD

"A long hot shower can be dangerous. The toxic chemicals are inhaled in high concentrations."

Is Your Water Safe—The Dangerous State of Your Water U.S. News & World Report, July 29,1991

http://www.holistichealthtools.com/chlorine.html

http://www.pubmedcentral.nih.gov/pagerender.fcgi?artid=1616111&pageindex=1

> **Comment:** The French do not drink chlorinated water. They ozonate their water to purify it. Ozonated water generally has a pH level of 8 (see chapter on pH).

The French are thought to have lower cancer rates by consuming high amounts of antioxidants such as oligomeric procyanidolic complexes (OPCs) and resveratrol found in red wine, which has made red wine famous for its health benefits. There is another side to their lower cancer rates that most people don't consider—ozonated water.

Does this make a difference? Absolutely.

According to the Medical College of Wisconsin Research Team "We are quite convinced that there is an association between cancer and chlorinated water."

We do not use chlorine because it is safe; we use it because it is *cheap*. We essentially still pour bleach in our water before we drink it. The long-term effects of chlorinated drinking water are disastrous.

According to the U.S. Council of Environmental Quality, "Cancer risk among people drinking chlorinated water is 93% higher than among those whose water does not contain chlorine."

It may cause much heart disease too. Dr. Joseph Price wrote a highly controversial book in the late sixties titled *Coronaries/Cholesterol/Chlorine* and concluded that nothing can negate the incontrovertible fact that the basic cause of arteriosclerosis, heart attacks, and stroke is chlorine.

Dr. Price later headed up a study using chickens as test subjects, where two groups of several hundred birds were observed throughout their life span to maturity.

One group was given water with chlorine and the other without. The group raised *with* chlorine, when autopsied, showed some level of heart or circulatory disease in every specimen; the group *without* had no incidence of disease. The group without chlorine grew faster, larger, and displayed vigorous health.

This study was well received in the poultry industry and is still used as a reference today.

http://www.purewatergazette.net/chlorinationfox.htm

As a result, most large poultry producers use de-chlorinated water.

When chlorine is added to our water, it combines with other natural compounds to form chlorination byproducts or trihalomethanes (THMs). These highly carcinogenic chlorine byproducts *trigger the production of free radicals in the body*, causing cell damage.

"Although concentrations of these carcinogens (THMs) are low, it is precisely these low levels that cancer scientists believe are responsible for the majority of human cancers in the United States". The Environmental Defense Fund stated simply that chlorine is a pesticide, whose singular purpose is to kill living organisms. When we consume chlorine-contaminated water, it kills some part of us, destroying cells and tissue inside our body.

The highly regarded University of Minnesota researcher Dr. Robert Carlson, who works for the U.S. Environmental Protection Agency, summed it up by claiming, "the chlorine problem is similar to that of air pollution". And he added that "chlorine is the greatest crippler and killer of modern times!"

http://www.callacooler.com.au/chlorine.html

Breast cancer, which now affects one in every eight women in North America, has recently been linked to the accumulation of chlorine compounds in the breast tissue. A study carried out in Hartford, Connecticut, the first of its kind in North America, found that:

"Women with breast cancer have 50% to 60% higher levels of organochlorines (chlorination byproducts) in their breast tissue than women without breast cancer."

It is not just *drinking* chlorinated water that is the problem.

Up to two-thirds of our exposure to chlorine is due to inhalation of steam and skin absorption while showering. A warm shower opens up the pores of the skin and allows for accelerated absorption of chlorine and other chemicals in water.

The steam we inhale while showering can contain up to *fifty times* the level of chemicals than tap water due to the fact that chlorine and most other contaminants vaporize much faster at a lower temperature than water. Inhalation is a much more harmful means of exposure since the chlorine gas (chloroform) we inhale goes directly into our bloodstream.

"Showering is suspected as the primary cause of elevated levels of chloroform in nearly every home because of chlorine in the water."

Dr. Lance Wallace, U.S. Environmental Protection Agency

http://www.cancerfightingstrategies.com/toxins.html

> **Comment:** Chlorine has seven electrons in its outer shell. This makes it reactive. Reactive elements are one electron short of a complete outer shell, and therefore, they are free radicals. Chlorine is a free radical and is very bad for us. The only way to remove it from our water is through filtration. Thus, another means of achieving and/or maintaining good health in the cancer equation is to remove chlorine from your diet.

CHAPTER 15

Why Fluoride is Your Enemy

Comment: Fluoride is like putting a corrosive poison in your humidifier. In Europe, the general public demanded the removal of fluoride from their water and succeeded! There are many places in the world that do not use fluoride, and in these places, there are very few cases of cavities!

To manufacture fluoride, phosphate rock is mined from the earth. Then water and sulfuric acid are added to create phosphoric acid, which, in turn, gives off hydrogen fluoride. The mix is placed into an evaporation unit to cook. The heat drives off the fluoride. The vapors are trapped off the phosphoric acid, which is "black as tar." Then, the vapors are condensed to form fluoride, also known as fluosilicic acid, hydrofluosilicic acid or sodium fluorosilicate.

Fluoride is second in toxicity to arsenic and more toxic than lead. Fluoride attaches to things like aluminum, metals and sodium.

Fluoride also is able to cross the blood brain barrier!

http://www.alternativesmagazine.com/17/green.html

"Cancer of the thyroid has been linked to highly fluoridated water."

Healthy Healing, Tenth Ed., Winner of Best Alternative Health Book 1998, p. H339

"Sodium fluoride acts as an internal poison to insects, and is frequently used in poison baits for Cockroaches, Earwigs, and other pests."

Bailliere's Encyclopedia of Scientific Agriculture, 1931, p. 601

"Fluoride is the only site contaminant which may cause adverse health effects to workers. Fluoride levels can result in an increase in the incidence of dental caries (or cavities) and skeletal fluorosis."

Quote from Agency for Toxic Substances and Disease Registry (ATSDR): "After entering your body, about *half* of the fluoride leaves the body quickly in urine, usually within 24 hours *unless large amounts (20 mg or more*, which is the amount in 20 or more liters of optimally fluoridated water) are ingested. Most of the fluoride ion that stays in your body is stored in your bones and teeth."

http://www.atsdr.cdc.gov/toxprofiles/phs11.html#bookmark05

> **Comment:** If I understand this correctly, if I drink two liters of water a day, in ten days I will have ingested a lethal quantity (20mg) of fluoride, only half of which will leave my body through urine (if I do not consume large amounts of water). So every day, I am supposed to drink one-tenth of a lethal dose of fluoride?

> *Did you know that* "fluoride, if consumed in concentrations greater than 1 parts per million (ppm) for extended periods of time can result in a dental condition known as *fluorosis*? Fluorosis, in severe cases, *can result in the deformation of the tooth enamel*, making it appear "mottled" with brown pits.

http://www.twinbrookdental.com/BJDfaq.htm

> **Comment:** You may not be aware but the U.S. Environmental Protection Agency determined that the maximum amount of fluoride allowed in drinking water is 4.0 milligrams per liter (mg/L).

http://www.atsdr.cdc.gov/toxprofiles/phs11.html#bookmark05

> **Comment:** Four milligrams! That is four times the optimal dose of fluoride that the government suggests or one fifth of a lethal dose of fluoride every day! Are we to believe that the government authorities are measuring the fluoride doses and testing the water for us, and that they never make mistakes, so we must be safe?

As of November 4th 2008, over 2,100 professionals urge the U.S. congress to stop water fluoridation until Congressional hearings could be conducted, citing scientific evidence that fluoridation, long promoted to fight tooth decay, is, in fact, ineffective and has serious health risks. Fifty-three U.S. cities rejected fluoridation that election day.

A study in rats and mice found that a small number of male rats developed bone cancer after drinking water with high levels of fluoride in it throughout their lives. This was considered *equivocal evidence that fluoride causes cancer* in male rats.

The International Agency for Research on Cancer (IARC) determined that the carcinogenicity of fluoride to humans is *not classifiable*. But, sodium fluoride, hydrogen fluoride, and fluorine are classified as "*hazardous substances*" by the Environmental Protection Agency.

http://www.atsdr.cdc.gov/toxprofiles/phs11.html#bookmark05

Studies based upon the U.S. Vital Statistics for fluoridated versus non fluoridated U.S. cities indicate a significant increase in cancer death rates occurring within the first two years of artificial fluoridation (greater than 99% confidence level). The nine organ sites affected and their increase above the normal are as follows:

Mouth, 15%;
Esophagus, 48%;
Stomach, 22%;
Large intestine, 31%;
Rectum, 51%;
Kidney, 10%;
Bladder and other urinary organs, 22%;
Other organs, specifically in women:
Breast, 15%; and
Ovary and fallopian tube, 15%.

Patients having cancers of these organ sites should be advised that they should not continue to drink or cook with fluoridated city water but should substitute bottled spring water or distilled water.

http://www.whale.to/d/fluoride.html

In 1992, a study on cancer by the New Jersey Department of Health in the United States found a strong link between fluoridation and bone cancer (osteosarcoma) in young males. They reported that the incidence of osteosarcoma was three to seven times higher in fluoridated areas than in non fluoridated areas.

http://www.thetruthseeker.co.uk/article.asp?ID=780

> **Comment:** Most people that I speak with about fluoride are not aware that the first use of fluorinated drinking water was in Germany, specifically in Nazi Prison camps. Their alleged reason for mass medication of water with sodium fluoride was "to sterilize humans and force the people into calm submission."

The Crime and Punishment of I.G. Farben, by Joseph Borkin

> **Comment:** Fluoride is added to almost all bottled water! So long story short, we need to be drinking filtered water. This is the only way to get rid of the toxic chlorine and fluoride from the water (which represents a significant portion of your body). Fluoride and chlorine cause cancer. If you want to be healthy or win a battle against cancer, I strongly suggest you address these issues as well.

Chapter 16

Ionized Water: as Good as it Gets

Comment: Not only is ionized water cleaner, it is very good for detoxification. It is more easily absorbed into the body, and it is also alkaline. If you are fighting cancer, then detoxification and becoming more alkaline are a must (see chapters on pH and detoxification). My water ionizer at home not only filters chlorine and fluoride (and many other toxic substances) but also produces alkaline water with a pH of 10.5. I can taste and feel the difference. When dealing with cancer, ionized water is the best you are ever going to get. I should mention as well that ionized water also acts as an antioxidant.

Free Radicals and Antioxidants Review:

Normally, bonds do not split in a way that leaves a molecule with an odd, unpaired electron. But when weak bonds split, free radicals are formed. Free radicals are very unstable and react quickly with other compounds, *trying to capture the needed electron to regain stability*. Generally, free radicals attack the nearest stable molecule, "stealing" its electron. When the "attacked" molecule loses its electron, it becomes a free radical itself, thereby beginning a chain reaction. Once the process is started, it can cascade, resulting in the disruption of a living cell.

The vitamins C and E are thought to protect the body against the destructive effects of free radicals. *Antioxidants neutralize free radicals by donating one of their own electrons*, ending the electron "stealing" reaction. The antioxidant nutrients themselves do not become free radicals by donating an electron because *they are stable in either form*. They act as scavengers, helping to prevent cell and tissue damage that could lead to cellular damage and disease.

Comment: Having ionized water in your house is like having the freshest stream of water in the world passing right through your house.

A water ionizer does three things:

First, electrolysis splits the water molecule in half, thus, leaving us with two parts, an acidic (free radical) water and alkaline (antioxidant) water. This process of splitting water in half and subsequent reduced size also makes for much better absorption. Everyone knows that bloated feeling when you drink too much water. This can be avoided with a water ionizer.

Second, it forces the removal of toxins (like chlorine and fluoride). Some toxins get pushed into a filter and some adhere to the metal plates inside the machine. This process makes for much cleaner water.

Third, the excess "acidic" water is expelled through one tube, and the "alkaline" water is expelled through the main tube. This alkaline water is good for balance because most of the regular food we eat is acidic (see chapter on pH). I also have noticed that since purchasing my water ionizer, I can now literally taste the difference between alkaline and acidic beverages. And on the rare occasion that I drink city tap water, I can taste "something extra" that I do not believe should be there.

Comment: Here is a quick explanation of how ionized water acts as an antioxidant.

An atom that acquires an electrical charge is called an ionized atom or an ion. This happens when an atom gains or losses one or more electrons, thus, changing the electrical balance between the protons and the electrons.

Ionized atoms can be negatively or positively charged. (Negative ionized atoms are called anions; positive ionized atoms are called cations.) Virtually, all reactions in biological systems are ionic. Ions are essential to plant and animal life.

When electricity is applied to water, ionization occurs. This process is called *electrolysis.*

Electrolysis causes water to separate into its basic components, hydrogen and oxygen gas.

And so, water or H_2O looks like this:

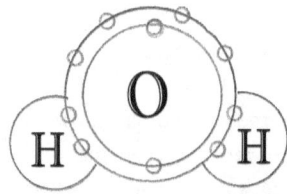

Water Molecule

During "electrolysis", two things are formed, "acid water" or hydronium ion and "alkaline water" or hydroxide ion.

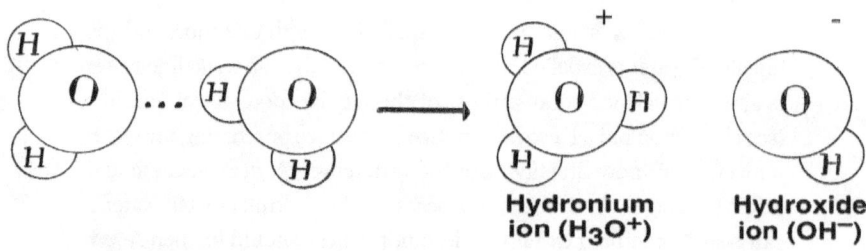

Hydronium
ion (H_3O^+)

Hydroxide
ion (OH^-)

HYDROXIDE ions have "the ability to *neutralize free radicals by donating one of their own electrons.* Thus, the antioxidant effects of ionized water, a.k.a. "alkaline water".

http://kentsimmons.uwinnipeg.ca/cm1504/water.htm

Comment: First, ionized water is cleaner.

Second, it is smaller and more easily absorbed.

Third, it is alkaline and has antioxidant properties. Since water represents more than half of your body mass, why not get the best water available? If you wish to be healthy or you are trying to fight cancer, I suggest very strongly that you start drinking ionized water.

CHAPTER 17

Your Friend The Sun

Comment: Almost all living things need sunlight to survive. The sun is the light in your home. Without it, you would stumble around your house like someone who has just lost his/her vision. It also is one of the most abundant sources of natural vitamin D available. A full spectrum of light is required for the conversion of cholesterol into vitamin D. This is inclusive of UVB rays, which are the same rays that cause cancer. Yes, the sun can prevent cancer and also cause cancer. The key is balance. If you overdo anything, it could cause cancer. However, you must have contact with the sun if you want to be healthy and avoid cancer.

THE SUN: Why Haven't You Heard about this Revolutionary Discovery?

If the sun *was* a drug, it would be hailed as the single greatest achievement of modern medical science. The developers would be the recipients of Nobel Prizes, and the story would be front-page news across the world. The patents would be worth many billions of dollars.

But that is just the thing. The substance that I am talking about is natural and freely available. It cannot be patented. Thus, there is almost no financial incentive for "modern medicine" to promote this life-saving substance. So guess what? They don't. Despite the fact that a groundbreaking new study showed that it could save nearly one million lives each year! In fact, the same study showed that six hundred thousand cases of breast and colon cancer alone could be prevented each year, if people simply increased their intake of this vital substance. Unfortunately, virtually 100% of the population is deficient in this substance at least part of the year according to several experts. That means there is a good chance that YOU are deficient. And there is no doubt that this will affect your health and longevity if you allow it to continue.

The miracle substance about which I am referring to is vitamin D. It is free of charge and available right outside your front door.

Your body is intricately designed to interact with the sun. You simply cannot function properly without it. Yet, we are constantly bombarded with so-called 'scientific' information to the contrary.

The message from dermatologists, medical professionals and other health authorities is nearly unanimous, "Stay out of the sun!" You have been told to keep indoors during peak sun hours and cover yourself with sunscreen when you do go outside.

All in the name of health.

But it may surprise you to learn that any evidence that exposing yourself to the sun is harmful evaporates under scrutiny. And if you follow this "no safe level of sun exposure" dogma, you could be putting yourself at greater risk of numerous deadly cancers, depression, bone loss, heart disease, diabetes, autoimmune illness, and a host of other ailments. In fact, even your risk of the deadly skin cancer melanoma could go up if you avoid spending time in the sun.

http://www.totalhealthbreakthroughs.com/ppc/sun-thankyou.html

> **Comment:** Could Seasonal Allergy Disorder (SAD) be related to lack of vitamin D? This next article states that vitamin D is an "assistant" to the signaling of cell death (such as cancer cell death).

Less Cancer in Those Closer to the Equator: More Sun, More Vitamin D, Less Cancer

In the July 2003 *Journal of Nutrition*, Jo Ellen Welsh of the University of Notre Dame and her colleagues reviewed the laboratory evidence on vitamin D and found that it signals breast, prostate, and colon cells to mature, stop growing, and to eventually succumb to programmed cell death or apoptosis. This is in contrast to cancer cells, which stay immature, keep growing and rapidly dividing, and do not die their natural death.

http://www.healthy-vitamins-rx.com/html/vitamin-d-deficiency.html

Vitamin D Deficiency

Osteomalacia is the general term for the softening of the bones due to defective bone mineralization. Osteomalacia in children is known as rickets, and because of this, osteomalacia is often restricted to the milder, adult form of the disease. It may show signs as diffuse body pains, muscle weakness, and fragility of the bones. A common cause of the disease is *a deficiency in vitamin D*, which is normally obtained from the diet and/or sunlight exposure.

http://en.wikipedia.org/wiki/Osteomalacia

> **Comment:** Many sunscreen agents, like octyl-methoxycinnamate, octyl-dimethylPABA (OD-PABA), benzophenone-3, homosalate (HMS), and 4-Methylbenzylidene camphor (4-MBC) are also endocrine disruptors, upsetting the body's hormone balance (discussed in later chapters). In particular, sunscreen agents have been shown to disrupt levels of estrogen, even allowing traces of their chemicals into breast milk. The higher the sun protector factor (SPF), the more toxic. Not surprisingly, there is a movement to outlaw any sunscreen with a SPF higher than 30.
>
> Would you eat sunscreen? You certainly would not after reading the poisonous contents in sunscreen. You should realize that what you put on your skin also goes directly into your body. This is yet another way to induce toxic overload in your system.
>
> Almost all the ads that tell you to stay out of the sun are put out by sunscreen companies. This becomes quite apparent when we become aware that 80% of these ads are in women's magazines. Women are the highest users of sunscreen. Again, these big companies profit from creating fear about the sun. It is all about the money!
>
> You do not require sunscreen. The proper response to the sun is lots of water, a proper dosing of vitamins, and a balanced amount of sun. Your skin is like a muscle that needs to be exercised to get stronger and more resilient. Your skin will need to get "exercised" in the sun. Then, as your skin gets stronger, it will be able to absorb more sun without being burned. Balance is the key. You need the sun to be healthy and prevent cancer. Removing it from the equation does not balance.

CHAPTER 18

Why You Need Vitamins and Essential Fats

Comment: Vitamins are like the framework of your house, the concrete base and the two-by-fours that hold up the frame. Vitamins and essential fats are yet another crucial piece of the equation that cannot be missing when fighting cancer. You need to know what it is that you are putting in your mouth. Information on food is another whole book onto itself, but let me just tell you that if your food comes in a can or box then it's probably not good for you. Things that are not good for you are usually bad for you. There is no in between.

Comment: Don't bother poisoning yourself with a multivitamin either. I could write a whole chapter on all the toxic materials, low-quality vitamins, and bonding agents that hold multivitamins together. These are what make them hard on your stomach and almost impossible to digest. Quality vitamins should be taken in liquid form on an empty stomach for best absorption.

In 1941, studies done by Dr. Agnes Faye Morgan at the University of California suggest that animals fed a synthetic vitamins-enriched diet had toxic reactions or died more quickly of degenerative diseases compared to those fed whole foods. She concluded that the enrichment of processed foods with synthetic vitamins may "precipitate conditions worse than the original deficiency."

Another 10-year study in twenty-nine thousand Finnish smokers supplemented with synthetic vitamins was stopped early because the death rates in the subjects given the synthetic vitamins was increased significantly;

namely, the risk of cancer increased by 16%, there were more heart attacks and strokes, and there was an 8% higher increase in the overall death rate.

A Harvard study in twenty-two thousand physicians reported no health benefits from synthetic vitamins. Other studies have reported increased toxicity and serious side effects. In one case, synthetic beta-carotene blocked antioxidant activity and the anticancer activity of fifty antioxidants in the diet.

In a Fred Hutchinson Cancer Research Center study, eighteen-thousand American men and women at risk of lung cancer were given either a placebo or a supplement of synthetic vitamin A. The investigators had to stop the study early because the group on synthetic vitamin supplements had a 28% higher incidence of lung cancer.

http://www.cancerfightingstrategies.com/other.html

> **Comment:** If the body is about balance, then unquestionably, we have to consider the simple things as well. Vitamins and essential fats to me are quite boring; however, you need to understand their importance in this "arch" that is good health. We also have to remember as well that without any probiotics in our bodies, we cannot digest food; and therefore, we cannot digest vitamins or minerals, and most nutrients will pass right through the body. All the pieces of this equation need to be working in conjunction with one another to help you deal with cancer.

About 74% of Americans ingest below the daily recommended daily allowance (RDA) requirements for magnesium, 55% are below for iron, 68% are below for calcium, 40% are below for vitamin C, 33% are below for vitamin B12, 80% are below for vitamin B6, 33% are below for vitamin B3, 35% are below for vitamin B2, 45% are below for vitamin B1, and 50% are below for vitamin A.

Twenty-five to 50% of hospital patients suffer from protein calorie malnutrition. Pure malnutrition (cachexia) is responsible for at least 22% and up to 67% of all cancer deaths. Up to 80% of all cancer patients have reduced levels of serum albumin, which is a leading indicator of protein and calorie malnutrition. At least 20% of Americans are clinically malnourished, with 70%

being sub clinically malnourished; and the remaining "chosen few" 10% are in good optimal health.

Patrick Quillin, PhD

http://www.whale.to/w/quotes4.html

> **Comment:** Remember I suggested earlier that *Candida* and cachexia are one and the same. *Candida* overgrowths will "steal" most of the vitamins you ingest for themselves, and without any good bacteria, very minimal amounts of vitamins will be digested; hence, the malnutrition of the "unexplained cachexia".

According to the *New York Times* (Aug 24, 2008), The body requires thirteen essential vitamins to function:

Vitamin A
Vitamin C
Vitamin D
Vitamin E
Vitamin K
Vitamin B1 (thiamine) Vitamin B2 (riboflavin)
Vitamin B3 (niacin)
Pantothenic acid
Biotin
Vitamin B6
Vitamin B12
Folate (folic acid)

These vitamins can be grouped into two categories: fat-soluble vitamins that are stored in the body's fatty tissue, and water-soluble vitamins that must be used by the body right away. Any leftover water-soluble vitamins leave the body through the urine. Vitamin B12 is the only water-soluble vitamin that can be stored in the liver for many years.

A.D.A.M. Inc.

Each vitamin has (a) specific function(s). You can develop health problems (e.g., deficiency disease) if you do not get enough of a particular vitamin.

Vitamin A helps in the formation and maintenance of healthy teeth, bones, soft tissue, mucous membranes, and skin.

Vitamin B6 is also known as *pyridoxine*. The more protein a person eats, the more vitamin B6 is needed to help the body use the protein. Vitamin B6 also helps form red blood cells and maintains brain function, among other things.

Vitamin B12, like the other B vitamins, is important for metabolism. It also helps to form red blood cells and maintain the central nervous system.

Vitamin C, also called *ascorbic acid*, is an antioxidant that promotes healthy teeth and gums. It helps the body absorb iron and maintain healthy tissue. It also promotes wound healing.

Vitamin D is also known as the *"sunshine vitamin"* since it is made by the body after being in the sun. This vitamin promotes the body's absorption of calcium, which is essential for the normal development and maintenance of healthy teeth and bones. It also helps maintain proper blood levels of calcium and phosphorus.

Vitamin E is an antioxidant also known as tocopherol. It plays a role in the formation of red blood cells and helps the body use vitamin K.

Vitamin K, which is not listed as an essential vitamin, is necessary for blood clotting (coagulation) that is important for vessel wall healing. Without vitamin K, individuals are at risk of excessive bleeding following injury. Some studies also suggest that vitamin K helps promote strong bones in the elderly.

Biotin is essential for the metabolism of proteins and carbohydrates and in the production of hormones and cholesterol.

Niacin is a B vitamin that helps maintain healthy skin and nerves. It also is thought to have some cholesterol-lowering effects.

Folate works with vitamin B12 to help form red blood cells. It is necessary for the production of DNA, which controls tissue growth and cell function. Any woman who is pregnant should be sure to get enough folate, since low levels of folate are linked to birth defects such as spina bifida. Many foods are now fortified with folic acid.

Pantothenic acid is essential for the metabolism of food. It also plays a role in the production of hormones and cholesterol.

Riboflavin (B2) works with the other B vitamins. It is important for body growth and the production of red blood cells.

Thiamine (B1) helps the body cells convert carbohydrates into energy. It also is essential for heart function and healthy nerve cells.

http://health.nytimes.com/health/guides/nutrition/vitamins/overview.html

> **Comment:** You need vitamin C for a myriad of body functions. Just to give you an idea how powerful a single vitamin can actually be, I direct your attention to the next article.

Vitamin C Injections Slow Tumor Growth in Mice

Researchers from the National Institutes of Health (NIH) investigated the anti-cancer effects of ascorbate on the formation of hydrogen peroxide in the extracellular fluid surrounding the tumors. High-dose injections of vitamin C, also known as ascorbate or ascorbic acid, reduced tumor weight and growth rate by about 50% in mouse models of brain, ovarian and pancreatic cancers. Normal cells were unaffected (published in the August 5, 2008, issue of the Proceedings of the National Academy of Sciences).

Natural physiologic controls precisely regulate the amount of ascorbate absorbed by the body when it is taken orally. "When you eat foods containing more than 200 milligrams of vitamin C per day, for example, two oranges and a serving of broccoli, your body prevents the blood levels of ascorbate from exceeding a narrow range," says Mark Levine, MD, the study's lead author and chief of the Molecular and Clinical Nutrition Section of the National Institute of Diabetes and Digestive and Kidney Diseases (NIDDK), part of the NIH. To bypass these normal controls, NIH scientists injected ascorbate into the veins or abdominal cavities of rodents with aggressive brain, ovarian, and pancreatic tumors. By doing so, they were able to deliver high doses of ascorbate, up to 4 grams per kilogram of body weight daily. "At these high injected doses, we hoped to see drug like activity that might be useful in cancer treatment," said Levine.

Then, they tested the effect(s) of ascorbate injections in immune-deficient mice with rapidly spreading ovarian, pancreatic, and glioblastoma (brain) tumors. The ascorbate injections reduced tumor growth and weight by 41 to 53%. In 30% of the/ glioblastoma placebo-treated animals, the cancer had spread to other organs, but in the ascorbate-treated animals, there were no signs of disseminated cancer. The investigators conclude that "These preclinical data provide the first firm basis for advancing pharmacologic ascorbate in cancer treatment in humans."

http://www.whale.to/a/vitctumour.html

> **Comment:** My understanding from these studies is that vitamin C kills tumors or retards tumor cell growth. Unfortunately, since your body has a mechanism that rigorously regulates a fixed amount of vitamin C absorption, it seems necessary that vitamin C should be injected directly into the blood stream or the tumor to bypass the body's own regulatory process.

Vitamin C Effects on Cancer Studies PubMed

http://www.pubmedcentral.nih.gov/articlerender.fcgi?artid=2596258&tool=pmcentrez

http://www.pubmedcentral.nih.gov/articlerender.fcgi?artid=2516245&tool=pmcentrez

http://www.pubmedcentral.nih.gov/articlerender.fcgi?artid=2516281

> **Comment:** You cannot take away any piece of this "arch" or your body will begin to break down. Essential fats are exactly that, namely, "essential". You need them to survive.

Essential Fats: Linoleic Acid (Omega-6) and Alpha-linolenic Acid (Omega-3)

Essential fats are not be made in the body. They are derived predominantly from vegetable oils and some omega-3s are derived from fish oils. These essential fats are needed for insulin metabolism (maintaining low body fat), oxygen uptake, regulation of blood pressure, and the formation of hemoglobin. They also form a major component of all cell membranes in your body.

Omega-3 and omega-6 essential fatty acids are part of the chain that makes three very important prostaglandins (short lived essential hormones). For example, prostaglandin E_1 (formed from alpha linolenic acid) and prostaglandin E_3 (formed from eicosapentaenoic acid) help stop blood platelets from sticking together. This is important in preventing blood platelet clots and subsequent heart attacks or strokes.

In contrast, prostaglandin E2 (derived from arachidonic acid), promotes platelet clumping, and is important for the function of your immune system, and in preventing dehydration.

Problem: Eating too much red meat and poor diets have skewed the ever so perfect balance of essential fat acid synthesis.

Solution: Eat less red meat and more fish, evening primrose, borage and black currant seed oil.

> **Comment:** There is no doubt that these are the basics of just being a normal healthy person. But if you are dealing with cancer, your body needs the boost of vitamins and essential fats. They are the "fuel" that your body runs on, and you will not get far without them. (Later chapters in this book will give you a few ways on how to get quality vitamins and essential fats into your diet).

CHAPTER 19

Why You Need Minerals

Comment: Minerals are like sheets of drywall in your house. You would not be complete without them. As I mention some basic facts on just a few minerals, you should begin to understand their relative importance in this equation we call "good health". Re-establishing good health is the only way that you can be free of cancer.

Minerals are the basic building blocks of all things, both living and nonliving. Their functions in our bodies are critical and are essential for good health.

The body utilizes over eighty minerals for maximum function. Because our plants and soils are so nutrient depleted, even if we eat the healthiest foods, we are not getting all the minerals we need. Evidence of mineral malnutrition is seen in various minor and serious health conditions such as energy loss, premature aging, diminished senses, and degenerative diseases like osteoporosis, heart disease and cancer.

In many cases, these can be prevented with proper mineral supplementation.

The more you learn about the benefits of minerals, the more you will be able to take charge of your own health!

Every living cell depends on minerals for proper structure and function. Minerals are needed for the formation of blood and bones, the proper composition of body fluids, healthy nerve function and proper operation of the cardiovascular system, among others. Like vitamins, minerals function as coenzymes, enabling the body to perform its functions including energy production, cell growth and healing. Because all enzyme activities involve minerals, they are essential for the proper utilization of vitamins and other nutrients. Nutritionally, minerals are grouped into two categories: bulk or essential minerals (also called macro minerals), and trace minerals or micro minerals. Macro minerals such as calcium and magnesium are needed by the body in larger amounts. Although only minute quantities of trace minerals are needed, they are nevertheless important for good health.

> **Comment:** Here is just a little information on a few macro minerals and their importance to good health.

Calcium

Calcium in the body must be tightly controlled because it is necessary for cell function for such things as blood clotting, muscle contraction, enzyme reactions, cellular communication and skin differentiation. It also gives bones and teeth their strength. In fact, the hardest substance in the human body, tooth enamel, is 95% calcium.

Calcium is rather deficient in the environment. The body has developed special mechanisms to extract calcium from dietary sources. Normal adults adapt to decreased calcium intake by increasing the fraction of dietary calcium absorbed, but absorption becomes retarded with aging. Some 30 to 60% of dietary intake is normally absorbed. Several hormones are involved in calcium metabolism. Two protein hormones, parathyroid hormone and calcitonin, and a derivative of vitamin D act to make sure the body optimally assimilates dietary calcium. A deficiency of calcium results in rickets in children and osteomalacia, both of which display a lack of bone mineralization. Calcium deficiency also may contribute to osteoporosis. Toxicity is rare except in certain diseases involving vitamin D or the parathyroid gland.

Dietary sources of calcium are mostly from the dairy foods. However, meat, some beans, seafood, tofu and green leafy vegetables contain substantial amounts of calcium. Seventy-two percent of the calcium available from dietary sources is normally consumed from the dairy group. An excellent calcium replacement for dairy products is soy (and soy products) and almond milk.

Phosphorus

Phosphorus is present in the body as inorganic phosphate or phosphate esters, which have many biological roles. Like calcium, the active form of vitamin D regulates phosphorus absorption. It is important for carbohydrate metabolism, cell membrane structure, transport processes, muscle function, and energy storage. Energy is stored in the form of adenosine triphosphate (ATP), which is used to fuel many biological processes. Phosphorus is present in nucleic acids and as a structural component of bones and teeth. The phosphate buffer system is important in maintaining the narrow pH range that is necessary for life.

Magnesium

Magnesium works in conjunction with many enzymes that are involved in energy metabolism, protein synthesis, and nucleic acid synthesis.

Many patients with migraine headaches have been found to have low levels of magnesium ions. Magnesium supplements appear to decrease the incidence of migraine attacks in certain people. Oral magnesium may be helpful in preventing premenstrual or menstrual migraines. It also may minimize premenstrual mood changes and fluid retention. When given intravenously (only under medical supervision), magnesium may be effective in treating cluster migraines.

Sodium

Sodium acts to maintain the normal hydration state of the bodily fluids. Sodium ions are found primarily in the plasma and fluid surrounding cells while potassium is found within cells. These ions affect the movement of water in an out of cells. Sodium ions balanced by other ions are necessary to normal cell function in all tissues of the body. Sodium may be involved in hypertension in some individuals.

Potassium

Potassium is essential to energy metabolism and to glycogen and protein synthesis. Because of its role in neuromuscular conduction, high or low levels of potassium can be life threatening. Too little potassium (hypoalemia) results in cardiac arrhythmias, muscle weakness, sodium loss in the urine, alterations in acid base balance, and the inefficient use of carbohydrate. Too much potassium (hyperkalemia) requires immediate medical attention because the heart may fail to beat normally or at all.

http://www.snyderhealth.com/minerals.htm

Comment: According to Everett Koop, former Surgeon General, *"Out of 2.1 million deaths a year in the United States, 1.6 million are related to poor nutrition."* Every little piece of this equation makes you stronger and stronger. If you are dealing with cancer, then it makes sense that you take all the help you can get. Minerals are essential to good health. Unfortunately, there is a very high probability that you are not getting enough of them. (Later on in this book, I will tell you some of the ways in which you can get proper amounts of minerals if you want to be healthy.)

CHAPTER 20

Melatonin (The Master Hormone) and Cancer

Comment: Hormones are yet another piece of the cancer/good health equation that we must consider. They must be balanced for your body to function properly. The next two chapters on hormones make me think of opening and closing the blinds in your house, predominantly because these two hormones relate to daytime and nighttime. One of these is melatonin, the nighttime hormone acts when the blinds are closed. I will only focus on two of several hormones to give you an idea of the importance of the roles that hormones play on our bodies in relation to cancer. If you understand how hormones play their parts, you may become more aware of the changes in your physical and/or mental well-being when their levels change in your body, and thus, you may be better informed on how to deal with any negative effects.

Comment on the Hormone Cascade: The key to understanding a hormone cascade is to understand that the top of the cascade is the controller for hormones farther downstream. For example, melatonin is the first hormone produced. Many hormones are produced after melatonin "downstream". Therefore, it is essential that the top hormone on the cascade (melatonin) starts everything off by being in sufficient supply.

Doctors have been using hormonal replacement therapies for the last three decades. But one of the problems is that they primarily replace the hormone that is low with a synthetic look alike hormone. At first glance, this approach seems logical. However, if we understand that the hormones in your body work like a teeter totter. When you add to one side of the beam, in order to maintain balance, you also must add to the other side of the beam. In actuality, this balance beam has many more than two arms, but for simplicity's sake, I digress. The point is, by simply replacing the one hormone that is deficient, does not address the issue concerning the underlying cause of that deficiency.

> **Comment:** For example, simply giving estrogen to someone low in estrogen may result in a disaster. Increasing estrogen itself can lead to an insufficiency and/or imbalance in testosterone, DHEA and progesterone. These sex-related hormones are linked together; replacing one changes the balance and sufficiency of the others. Thus, when estrogen is given, DHEA also may be needed. In addition, changes in testosterone and progesterone levels may need to be addressed as they may not remain in balance or are of insufficient supply. The message is that hormones need to be given in combination, which leads to feedback situations that aid in maintaining a healthy balance. This results in more stability within the hormonal cascade.

> **Comment:** Almost any naturopath can do hormone testing for you, but you also can mail a saliva sample to a number of laboratories that can test it for you.

According to investigators at the University of Maryland Medical Center, melatonin, "the master hormone" is the first hormone secreted by the pineal gland in the brain. Melatonin helps regulate other hormones that affect your emotions, muscles, bones, intelligence and immunity, and maintains the body's circadian rhythm. The circadian rhythm is an internal twenty-four timekeeping system that plays a critical role in determining when we fall asleep and when we wake up. Darkness stimulates the production of melatonin while light suppresses its activity. Exposure to excessive light in the evening or too little light during the day can disrupt the body's normal melatonin cycles. For example, jet lag, shift work, and poor vision will disrupt melatonin cycles. In addition, some experts claim that exposure to low-frequency electromagnetic fields (common to household appliances) may disrupt the normal cycles and production of melatonin (see chapter on EMFs).

Melatonin also helps control the timing and release of female reproductive hormones. Thus, it helps determine when menstruation begins, the frequency and duration of menstrual cycles, and when menstruation ceases (menopause).

> **Comment:** Menopause (known as andropause in men) happens when and because hormone production drops below normal adult

levels. For example, a drop in estrogen in one reason why the growth of a baby can no longer be supported in the female body after menopause.

Many researchers also suggest that melatonin levels are related to the aging process. Specifically, young children have the highest levels of nighttime melatonin. These levels diminish as we age. The decline in melatonin may explain why many older adults have disrupted sleep patterns and tend to go to bed and wake up earlier than when they were younger.

In addition to its hormonal actions, melatonin has strong antioxidant effects. Preliminary evidence suggests that it may help strengthen the immune system.

http://www.umm.edu/altmed/articles/melatonin-000315.htm

Comment: The normal melatonin cascade in adults over seventy years of age is summarized in the chart below.

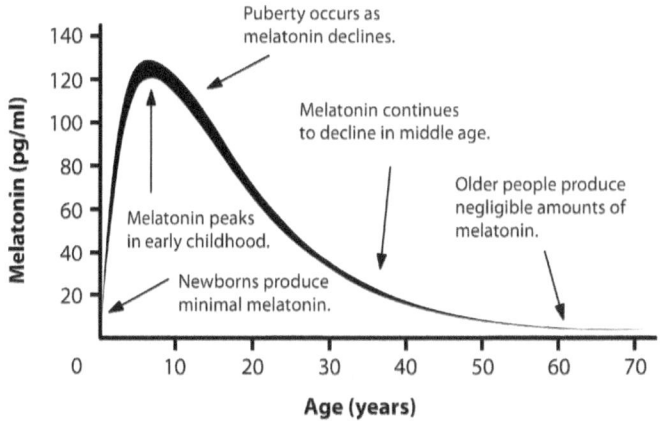

http://www.cocoonnutrition.org/catalog/NL_docs/melatoninnl_files/chart.jpg

Comment: According to Dr. Michael Colgan, numerous studies indicate that the disruption in circadian rhythm in shift workers increases their risk of cancer by about 300%. Keep in mind, on top of requiring the right balance of hormones to function properly, your body does most of its repairing when you sleep.

At McMaster University in Canada, researchers did a systematic review of studies related to melatonin in patients with solid tumor cancer and its effect on their survival at one year. From ten studies published between 1992 and 2003, they concluded that melatonin reduced the risk of death at one year, regardless of the type of cancer. Equally important, those studies suggested that there were no serious adverse effects.

Mills E, Wu P, Seely D, Guyatt G. Melatonin in the treatment of cancer: a systematic review of randomized controlled trials and meta-analysis. J Pineal Res, 2005; 39(4):360-6.

Saez MC, Barriga C, Garcia JJ et al. Melatonin increases the survival time of animals with untreated mammary tumors:

Neuroendocrine stabilization. Mol Cell Biochem. 2005; 278(1-2):15-20. Schernhammer ES, Hankinson SE. Cancer Inst. Urinary melatonin levels and breast cancer risk. J Nat Cancer Inst 2005; 97(14):1084-7.

http://altmedicine.about.com/od/cancer/a/melatonin_cance.htm

> **Comment on Seasonal Affective Disorder:** Light entering the eyes "shuts off" the use of melatonin. Consequently, staring at computer screens, watching television or trying to sleep is more difficult during the day with the extra light entering the eyes. This is a good reason why you should not to do these things before going to bed. Conversely, the lack of light will cause more melatonin production. This may be one of the explanations why people feel so tired in the winter. More darkness equates to more melatonin production.

"Melatonin is a potent immune-enhancing hormone produced by the human pineal gland and appears to have substantial cancer-repressing effects. In addition to enhancing the activity of key immune cells called T helper cells, melatonin stimulates the tumor-killing action of natural killer cells (NK) by increasing the white blood cell production of the cytokine Interleukin-2 (IL-2).

Definitive Guide to Cancer by John Diamond, MD and Lee Cowden, MD

Breast Cancer: Several studies indicate that melatonin levels may be linked with breast cancer risk. Women with breast cancer tend to have lower levels of melatonin than those without the disease. In addition, laboratory experiments have found that low levels of melatonin stimulate the growth of certain types of breast cancer cells, while adding melatonin to these cells inhibits their growth. Preliminary laboratory and clinical evidence also suggest that melatonin enhances the effects of some chemotherapy drugs used to treat breast cancer. In a study of a small number of women with breast cancer, melatonin (administered seven days before beginning chemotherapy) prevented the lowering of platelets in the blood. This is a common complication of chemotherapy, known as thrombocytopenia, can lead to bleeding.

In another study of a small group of women whose breast cancer was not improving with tamoxifen (a commonly used chemotherapy medication), adding melatonin resulted in a 28% decrease in tumors size.

Prostate Cancer: Like breast cancer, there have been studies that show that male patients with prostate cancer have lower melatonin levels than men without the disease. Melatonin also inhibits the growth of prostate cancer cells in test tube studies. In a small-scale study, melatonin (used in combination with conventional medical treatment) improved the survival rates in nine out of fourteen patients with metastatic prostate cancer. Interestingly, since meditation may cause melatonin levels to rise, meditation also may be a valuable adjunct to the treatment of prostate cancer.

Interleukin-2: In one study of eighty cancer patients, use of melatonin in combination with interleukin-2 led to more tumor regression and better survival rates than a treatment with interleukin-2 alone.

Cancer-related weight loss: Weight loss and malnutrition are concerns for people with cancer. In one study of one hundred people with advanced cancer, those who received melatonin supplements were less likely to lose weight than those who did not receive the supplements.

> **Comment:** If you only sleep for a few hours a night, your body will require more food and energy to function during the extended hours of wakefulness. This is especially true if you have a cancer tumor somewhere in your body because cancer is fast growing and consumes a tremendous proportion of your body's total energy.

Other substances such as caffeine, tobacco and alcohol can diminish the levels of melatonin in your body while cocaine and amphetamines may increase melatonin production.

http://www.umm.edu/altmed/articles/melatonin-000315.htm

Comment: Melatonin was considered an "illegal" substance in Canada until about 1996.

Comment: You make most or all of your red blood cells in the first two hours of sleep. Perhaps this is the reason why "power" naps make you feel like you have been 'recharged'; e.g., naps = new blood cells + rest and repair.

If you prefer to keep it simple, just remember this, if you do not have any melatonin, you cannot sleep. If you do not sleep, your immune system will not work effectively and your body will not repair itself. Without an effective repair process, you will most likely get sick and increase your risk of developing cancer. So get a regular amount of sleep!

CHAPTER 21

DHEA
(Dehydroepiandrosterone)
and Cancer

Comment: Like a gas pedal and a clutch that must be balanced, melatonin is the counterbalance to DHEA. DHEA is the daytime hormone used for many things including cognitive function. Since it is stimulated by light entering the eyes, I think of DHEA as "having the blinds in your house open". This was of some concern to me after my kidney (and adjacent adrenal gland, another key hormone producer) were removed. I ended up with having daily and quite severe mental exhaustion between 2:00 and 4:00 PM. My cognitive function (not my energy) would drop to about 30 to 40%. I also would lose coordination and become lightheaded or dizzy. However, once I had a two hour nap, I would wake up feeling better than I did the first thing in the morning. I concluded that these episodes were due to an interruption in my hormonal cascade, such as not producing enough DHEA, which, in turn, resulted in a loss of cognitive function, coordination, and mental tiredness.

In order to assess how DHEA affects good health and cancer, first, we need to know a little about DHEA.

Very Brief Abstract of Theory: In daytime concentrations, DHEA acts with specific proteins as the molecule of consciousness, i.e., it enhances the activation of the nervous system. During deep sleep, the concentrations of DHEA are reduced such that only enough DHEA is produced to maintain autonomic functions. The production of melatonin, the molecule for sleep, is reduced when the production of DHEA increases. During sleep, reduced nighttime levels of DHEA reciprocate with melatonin to produce either slow-wave sleep (SWS) or rapid eye movement (REM) sleep. These low productions of DHEA are higher during REM sleep and lower during SWS. During sleep, melatonin becomes consumed or "used up", allowing for an increased production of DHEA. In contrast, during consciousness, DHEA is consumed and melatonin production increases, but it is not released until the DHEA levels have declined to the low levels prior to sleep.

http://www.anthropogeny.com/Sleep%20and%20SIDS.htm

DHEA is a natural sterone or ketone derived from a steroid, and is produced naturally in the body by the adrenal glands. DHEA is the sole precursor and regulator for the natural production of every steroid and sex hormone in the body. It does this by the conversion of cholesterol. Specifically, DHEA is necessary for the body to produce healthy levels of all the other hormones required for healthy body function. DHEA is the most common sterone in human blood. These sex hormones and their metabolites can promote cell proliferation (an increase in the number of cells as a result of cell growth and cell division). DHEA is known as the mother hormone because it is the primary hormone and precursor to all other hormones. Research indicates that the younger you are the more DHEA you have. It is the primary indicator of youth and also known as the *"youth hormone"*.

The aging process is inextricably tied to a decrease in beneficial hormones, such as growth hormone, thyroid, and DHEA. An increase in hormones to excess levels is clearly harmful, such as insulin that regulates glucose levels and cortisol, a stress hormone. One of the primary changes felt with aging is fatigue. The loss of energy in the late afternoon, the decrease in productivity at work, the inability to exercise due to exhaustion, and the feeling of unrest after a fitful night's sleep, all are related to the aging process. As such, one may sense a feeling of frustration associated with becoming short tempered, being unable to concentrate, and growing intolerant to change. DHEA seems to be a key to understanding this fatigue that occurs with aging. DHEA is necessary for the production of energy as it drives the energy producing parts of the cells.

DHEA also is vital to burning fat. That is why along with fatigue, elderly individuals often gain weight and store the fat particularly in the abdominal region. Additional fat deposits also are accumulated around the heart and in the blood vessels, the latter contributing to the development of arteriosclerosis. Thus, a supplement of DHEA to replace that lost in the aging process, may improve his or her energy level. And with subsequent renewed energy, an older person may become better able to exercise and more easily adopt life style that may lead to a decreased risk in some of these diseases associated with limited or no physical activities. The current medical literature suggests that select patient populations with chronic complaints of fatigue, headache, obesity, and depression have low DHEA blood levels comparable to the DHEA levels seen in very old individuals. Could this explain why these patients are relatively unable to function? It may further illustrate what a lack of energy does to the body's systems; namely, it weakens the immune system, thereby inhibiting the body's ability to fight infection.

Research suggests that there is a significant correlation between low DHEA levels and a impaired immune system. DHEA is now being used in the fight against HIV, cancer, and senile dementia. Clinically, it has been shown that DHEA helps brain neurons establish contact. Furthermore, it is known that Alzheimer patients have low DHEA levels when compared to their healthy counterparts. The amount of DHEA the body produces drops dramatically as people age. When the average person reaches seventy years of age, his/her body only produces about 10% of the DHEA that a twenty-five year old produces. This may explain why many medical researchers believe that reestablishing the levels of DHEA seen in the younger population may be an important step in achieving 'natural' antiaging.

The dramatic drop in DHEA levels observed during aging parallels the development of degenerative syndromes such as immune senescence, atherosclerosis, osteoporosis, cognitive decline, depression, and increased risk of cancer. The elderly suffer from a decline in DHEA secretion and a rise in cortisol. Those with very low levels of DHEA and higher levels of cortisol are most likely to suffer from dementia. The neuroprotective effects of DHEA replacement may be the most important antiaging benefit, since ultimately there is nothing as important as slowing down the aging of the brain.

http://womens-health.health-cares.net/anti-aging-dhea.php

Comment: The DHEA cascade of people over eighty years of age is shown in the chart below.

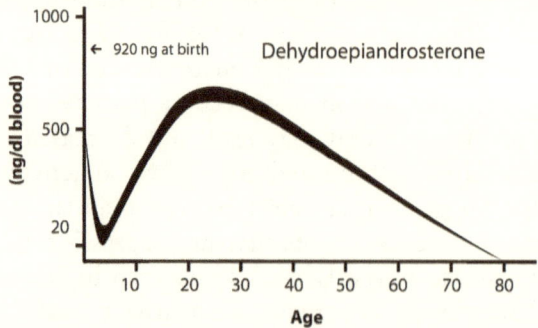

http://cellfood.microwaterman.com/images/CellFood/dhea_chart.gif

In women, DHEA is the first hormone to decline significantly with peri menopause, at about age of thirty-five years, thereby starting the downward spiral into the degenerative condition of menopause.

Colgan M. Hormonal Health. Vancouver, BC: Apple Publishing, 1996

Unless DHEA levels are at least at the level of an average thirty-year old, all of the typical fat loss schemes that manipulate food and exercise can achieve only short-term results. Therefore, they are doomed to repeated failure that makes fat loss progressively more difficult. That, in turn, can promote degenerative disease. Daily low dose DHEA supplementation is a key variable in prevention.

http://www.vistamagonline.com/articles/page.php?tp=1&p=3&id=14&s=the_deal _with_the_dhea

DHEA and Cancer

Early reports from England (Bulbrook, 1962, 1971) suggest that DHEA is abnormally low in women who develop breast cancer, even as much as nine years prior to the onset or diagnosis of the disease. Five thousand of these women were followed in the study. Twenty-seven women developed cancer. Most of these had abnormally low levels of DHEA. If low DHEA levels contributed to breast cancer, it could be argued that the opposite is true. Consistent with that possibility, Dr. Arthur Schwartz and colleagues at Temple University found that a supplement of DHEA significantly protected cell cultures from the toxicity of carcinogens. Cell cultures usually respond to powerful carcinogens with mutations (changes in DNA), transformations (changes in cell appearance), and a high rate of cell death. But when DHEA was added with the carcinogen, all three of these responses were decreased significantly.

DHEA is known to enhance general immune response. Oral and subcutaneous (injected) DHEA have been observed to protect rodents against the lethality of RNA and DNA viruses and lethal bacterial infections.

Because of its generally universal function in human metabolism, DHEA is being associated with numerous human maladies. For example, DHEA has recently been found to have a highly statistically significant correlation with vertebral bone density in postmenopausal women, suggesting that DHEA (and other weak androgens) may protect against osteoporosis.

http://www.ceri.com/dhea.htm

It is also known that a small amount of sulphate DHEA and micronized DHEA is converted into testosterone. DHEA is most overlooked but its vital role may be its relationship with cortisol. Recent research indicates that DHEA has an inverse relationship with cortisol, e.g., when DHEA is low, cortisol levels are high, and vice-versa. Cortisol is one of the few hormones that increase with age; it is known to induce stress, and when allowed to circulate at high levels for long periods, may affect many body functions, including insulin resistance and damage to the endocrine system via damage to the hypothalamus. Maintaining healthy levels of DHEA for aging and stressed individuals may be important because of DHEA's ability to help lower cortisol levels.

http://www.biogenesis.co.za/pi-dhea.asp

> **Comment:** I can verify personally that DHEA counterbalances to cortisol. In the past, when I became very stressed, I felt like I was going to pass out. I never actually did pass out, but I was unable to think clearly (lack of DHEA?) and had a difficult time trying to "calm down" (leftover adrenalin). This becomes easy to understand when we consider one of the main effects of stress is adrenalin. The only way to break down the "leftover" adrenalin (that does not get used up) is with cortisol, which is one counterbalance to DHEA! More stress and adrenalin in your body equates to more cortisol, which, in turn, depletes DHEA, thereby affecting cognitive function!

> **Comment on Rainy Days and Shift Work:** Did you know that DHEA production is induced by light entering the eyes? Could

this be the reason that sales, the number of road crashes, and the general attitude of the public is affected on rainy days? Could this be the reason that night shift workers (who have difficulty regulating hormone balance, a problem induced by abnormal sleep and light cycles affecting circadian rhythms, have a 300% increase in the probability of cancer? They do not produce enough melatonin (inducing sleep and repair) during the day with all the light. Their bodies are never "told" (through absence of light) to make DHEA when they are awake at night.

CHAPTER 22

Why You Need Glutamine

Comment: There are twenty amino acids that we know of and nine of these are thought to be essential for orderly body function (there is that word "*essential*" again). Amino acids are the screws, nails, nuts, and bolts that hold the house together. Without them, all the other pieces in the house just barely hold together. I mention only two amino acids because this book is not supposed to be a dictionary of health. It is only supposed to give you an introductory understanding of how all the building blocks of your body fit and work together. When you understand that, you will understand how to prevent and reverse cancer.

Comment: Glutamine is the most abundant amino acid in the body and is involved in many metabolic processes. Amino acids are yet another piece of the equation that is cancer.

Glutamine is an amino acid that helps build and maintain the muscles of the body. It also helps to remove toxic ammonia from the liver and to maintain a healthy central nervous system.

Glutamine is in high demand throughout the body. It is used in the gut and immune system extensively to maintain optimal performance. Glutamine plays a very important role in protein metabolism and synthesis as well as optimizing normal brain function and digestion. It is able to cross the blood brain barrier and becomes glutamic acid, an important brain fuel. Glutamine helps maintain cell volume and hydration, enhances wound and burn healing time. It also is one of the most important nutrients for your intestines. It has the ability to maintain the structural integrity of bowels. Glutamine is important for removing excess ammonia (a common waste product in the body). Depleted glutamine stores make it nearly impossible to recover properly from heavy workouts. Your body is thrown into a catabolic state in which it is cannibalizing its own muscle for the building materials for glutamine. Your body needs glutamine more than it needs the extra muscle!

During heavy activity, it can be depleted more than 40%, which, in turn, will drastically impair energy and suppress the immune system. Your body will struggle to replace lost glutamine by consuming branched chain amino acids out of the skeletal muscle tissue to reconstruct glutamine molecules.

http://www.bodybuilding.com/fun/mdlabs12.htm

Glutamine promotes normal cell division throughout the body. It is key to the development of DNA and RNA, and to the formation of cells that function as part of the immune system, such as thymocytes, lymphocytes, and macrophages. Without sufficient glutamine, the immune system would cease to function. For this reason, glutamine is sometimes recommended for people who suffer from diseases linked to the malfunctioning of the immune system, such as rheumatoid arthritis, chronic fatigue, scleroderma and AIDS. Glutamine also may be useful to those recovering from surgery or acute injury when the body is under stress. When under stress, the body may release as much as one-third of the glutathione into muscles to provide extra fuel to the injury site, and supplementation may be necessary to prevent muscle cannibalization.

http://www.vitaminstuff.com/glutamine.html

Glutamine and Cancer

Many people with cancer have abnormally low levels of glutamine. For this reason, some experts speculate that glutamine may prove to be a good adjunct to conventional cancer therapy under certain conditions. In fact, nutritional support with supplemental glutamine is often used in malnourished cancer patients undergoing chemotherapy or radiation treatments and sometimes used in patients undergoing bone marrow transplants.

Glutamine is used to protect the lining of the small and large intestines from damage caused by chemotherapy or radiation. Glutamine also may protect against the development of mucositis (breakdown of the mucosal membranes of the mouth and nasal passages) caused by therapy for head and neck cancer.

Wound Healing

When the body is stressed (such as from injuries, infections, burns, trauma, or surgical procedures), steroid hormones such as cortisol are released into the bloodstream. Elevated cortisol levels can deplete glutamine stores in the body. Since glutamine plays a key role in the immune system, a deficiency in this nutrient can significantly slow the healing process. Studies have shown that glutamine supplements enhance the immune system and reduce infections (particularly infections associated with surgery). Glutamine supplements also may aid in the recovery of severe burns.

Inflammatory Bowel Disease (IBD)

Glutamine helps to protect the lining of the gastrointestinal tract known as the mucosa. Because of this, some experts speculate that glutamine deficiency may play a role in the development of IBD, namely ulcerative colitis and Crohn's disease. These conditions are characterized by damage to the mucosal lining of the small and/or large intestines, which leads to inflammation, infection, and ulcerations (holes). In fact, some preliminary research suggests that glutamine may be a valuable supplement during treatment of IBD because it promotes healing of the cells in the intestines and improves diarrhea associated with IBD. However, not all studies have found this positive benefit. Consequently, more research is needed before any conclusions can be drawn. In the meantime, follow the advice of your healthcare provider when deciding whether to use glutamine for IBD.

http://www.umm.edu/altmed/articles/glutamine-000307.htm

In a recent study of the role of glutamine in enhancing the immune system, investigators found that increased levels of glutamine leads to greater amounts of virus and infection fighting cells, T and B Lymphocytes.

Hankard RG, Haymond MW, Darmaun D. Effect of glutamine on leucine metabolism in humans. Am J Physiol, 1996; 271:E748-54).

Studies indicate that low levels of glutamine may be associated with increased susceptibility to infections and illness due to a suppressed immune system.

Castell LM, Poortmans JR, Newsholme EA. Does glutamine have a role in reducing infections in athletes? Eur J Appl Physiol, 1996; 73: 488-90.

> **Comment:** Glutamine is the most abundant amino acid in the body. It is involved with the removal of toxic ammonia, maintaining a healthy central nervous system, protein metabolism and protein

synthesis. It also promotes normal cell division, only to name a few things. It is in high demand for proper body function, which is why it is an "essential" amino acid. If you are attempting to deal with cancer or just to be healthy, need to have enough of amino acids (including glutamine).

CHAPTER 23

Why You Need L-Arginine

Comment: L-arginine is another amino acid that is a substantial part of this equation that is good health. You need it, along with several other amino acids to facilitate proper body functions.

Arginine is a semi essential amino acid. It is a building block of protein that performs a myriad of physiological functions. It is a known precursor of the gas nitric oxide (NO2). (Nitric oxide controls vessel wall caliber and transmits messages between nerve cells).

Arginine is an amino acid that the body cannot make naturally. Therefore, it is important to consume foods that are rich in arginine.[1]

Arginine is found in high concentrations in nuts and seeds like peanuts and almonds. It also is found in chocolate and raisins.

Arginine is necessary for the execution of many physiological processes. These physiological processes include hormone secretion, an increase in growth hormone output, the removal of toxic waste products from the body, and immune system defenses.[2]

Because arginine is a precursor of nitric oxide (which regulates vasodilatation or the expansion of cells[3]), it is often used for supporting healthy sexual function.

Recently, dietary supplements containing arginine have become popular due to arginine's nitric oxide producing ability, its ability to scavenge free radicals, as well as its ability to signal muscle cells, release growth hormone, support healthy cholesterol, and enhance fat metabolism. Arginine helps regulate salt levels in the body.[4]

Arginine also is thought to be crucial for muscle growth due to its vasodilating abilities, as well as its ability to participate in protein synthesis.[5]

1. Alternative Medical Review. 2002, Dec 7 (6): 512-22.
2. Appleton, J. Arginine: Clinical potential of a semi-essential amino. Altern Med Rev, 2002; 7(6):512-522.
3. Nakaki T, Kato R. 1994. Beneficial circulatory effect of L-arginine. Jap J Pharmacol, Oct, 66 (2): 167-71.
4. *http://1001herbs.com/l-arginine/*
5. Reyes AA, Karl IE, Klahr S. Role of arginine in health and in renal disease [editorial] Am J Physiol, 1994; 267: 3 Pt 2, F331-46.

http://www.bodybuilding.com/store/arginine.html

Wound healing

The effect of L-arginine on wound repair may be associated with its role in the formation of L-proline, an important amino acid essential for the synthesis of collagen.

Other Conditions

L-arginine also is used for high blood pressure, migraines, sexual dysfunction in women, intermittent claudication, and interstitial cystitis.

Erectile Dysfunction

L-arginine has been used for erectile dysfunction. Like the drug sildenafil citrate (Viagra), L-arginine is thought to enhance the action of nitric oxide, which relaxes muscles surrounding blood vessels supplying the penis. As a result, blood vessels in the penis dilate, increasing blood flow, which helps maintain an erection. Viagra maintains an erection by blocking an enzyme called PDE5, which destroys nitric oxide, whereas L-arginine facilitates the production of nitric oxide.

http://altmedicine.about.com/cs/herbsvitaminsad/a/Arginine.htm

> **Comment:** Notice that L-arginine relaxes muscles and is used for migraines (see chapter on oxygen and migraines).

Arginine Deficiency

Symptoms of arginine deficiency include poor wound healing, hair loss, skin rash, constipation, and fatty liver, insomnia, un-refreshing sleep, lack of dreaming, prostate enlargement, cataracts and high blood pressure.

L-arginine is needed to create urea, a waste product that is necessary for toxic ammonia to be removed from the body. In 1939, researchers discovered that L-arginine also is needed to make creatine, a nitrous organic acid that also facilitates muscle growth. Creatine breaks down into creatinine at a constant rate, and then it is cleared from the body by the kidneys.

http://www.mayoclinic.com/health/l-arginine/NS_patient-arginine

> **Comment:** L-arginine plays a role in hormone secretion, growth hormone output, the removal of toxic wastes, and immune system defenses. It is a precursor to nitric oxide, a scavenger of free radicals, a regulator of salts and protein synthesis, only to name a few things. I hope you are starting to see now that if even one of these building blocks in your body is out of place, then the whole body begins to get weaker. If you are trying to be healthy or fighting cancer, then you also need to pay attention to amino acids, two of which are glutamine and L-arginine. Other major building blocks of your body are discussed in the chapter on *Spirulina*.

Chapter 24

Psychological Mindset: Your Mind Controls Your Body

Comment: If you plan on beating cancer, you also need to get your mindset in the right place. Being stressed out or emotionally upset is like living in a haunted house with monsters chasing you. It becomes difficult to concentrate on anything else. In order for our minds and bodies to be at peace, we need to live in a house with soothing colors and beautiful artwork. Your heart, for example, is operating because of subconscious signals from your brain. Therefore, *"your mind controls your body"*.

Comment: Stomach aches, back pain, neck cramps—we all know stress causes a disruption in the body's internal signals. Personally, I have given myself a migraine in less than ten minutes just from being stressed. It is unquestionable that how we feel inside has an effect on our bodies. But what effect? A good example of just how effectively your mind controls your body is the "fight-or-flight" response. The "fight-or-flight" stress response involves a cascade of biological changes that prepares us for emergency action in response to danger. When danger is sensed, a small part of the brain called the hypothalamus sets off a chemical alarm. The sympathetic nervous system responds by releasing a flood of stress hormones, including adrenaline, norepinephrine and cortisol. These stress hormones race through the bloodstream, preparing us to either flee the scene or fight it out.

http://www.employeesfirst.ie/resources/documents/StressUnderstandingStress.doc

Comment: The fight-or-flight response starts first in the brain with fear. It is an emotion created internally by our perception of the external environment. Therefore, our perception of the outside environment can have dramatic effects on our internal systems. This is known as the autonomic nervous system (ANS), which is the part of the nervous system in charge of regulating *involuntary* vital functions, including the activity of the heart, the digestive system and the glands. It can be divided into two subsystems, the sympathetic nervous system and the parasympathetic nervous system. The sympathetic nervous system responds to stress by speeding up the heart rate, constricting blood vessels and decreasing digestive activity in the intestines and increasing blood pressure, thereby preparing the body to either fight or flee (the fight-or-flight response). In contrast, parasympathetic nervous system counteracts the sympathetic nervous system response by slowing down the heart rate, increasing blood flow in the digestive tract, and relaxing muscles.

http://stress.about.com/od/stressmanagementglossary/g/ans.htm

Comment: An example of how stress causes sickness is illustrated by the following study.

A group of researchers at the Garvan Institute in Sydney reported that the hormone, known as neuropeptide Y, is released into the body during times of stress. Neuropeptide Y can inhibit the immune system from functioning properly. Neuropeptide Y increases blood pressure and heart rate, but it is not known whether it actually affects immune cells as well.

These investigators concluded that there is a direct link, and that stress not only can weaken the immune system but also makes you more vulnerable when, for example, you have a cold or flu and even in the more serious situations such as cancer can be enhanced in these situations.

http://www.abc.net.au/news/newsitems/200512/s1523294.htm

Stress also can significantly increase the transport of chemicals across the blood brain barrier. During the Gulf War, Israeli soldiers were given a drug called pyridostigmine to protect themselves from chemical and biological weapons. Normally, pyridostigmine does not cross the blood brain barrier. However, almost one-quarter of the soldiers who took the drug complained of headaches, nausea, and dizziness, symptoms associated with pyridostigmine if and when it actually crosses the blood brain barrier. It was concluded that the stress of war had somehow increased the permeability of the blood brain barrier, although the explanation for this stress induced change in the permeability of the blood brain barrier is not entirely clear. Nonetheless, these observations have significant implications since they demonstrate that stress can have a significant effect that may result in unexpected effects of certain drugs, which under other conditions are thought NOT to cross blood brain barrier.

http://www.fi.edu/learn/brain/stress.html

Stress Can Make You Sick, But It Does Not Have To.

Studies suggest that people with medical conditions such as heart disease, mental illness or other chronic diseases, are most vulnerable to the negative consequences of stress, but it should be noted that healthy people when stressed also are at a risk.

The link between stress and heart-related problems has been widely studied. Evidence also suggests that mental stress increases the body's demand for oxygen when blood pressure and heart rate are increased. For people who have suffered a previous heart disease, this additional burden can result in an increase risk of a second heart attack or stroke, and even death.

Stress also can act as a trigger for heart attack or stroke in people with undiagnosed heart disease, according to David S Krantz, PhD, chairman of the department of medical and clinical psychology at Uniformed Services University in Bethesda, MD. He suggested that stress can result in dangerous plaque ruptures in people who may not know that they are in the early stages of atherosclerosis or "hardening" of the arteries. These plaque ruptures can lead to potentially life-threatening events like heart attacks or strokes.

Steven Tovian PhD, director of health psychology at Evanston Northwestern Health Care Center in Evanston, IL suggested that stress also directly affects the part of the nervous system that regulates glandular, heart, digestive, respiratory and skin function.

These observations suggest that many pre-existing medical conditions, which are influenced by a nervous system response, such as chronic pain, irritable bowel syndrome (IBS), digestive disorders, and headaches, also are likely to become exacerbated by stress when the already overworked system becomes overloaded by additional stress.

Jennifer Warner, WebMD Feature reviewed by Charlotte Grayson

http://www.medicinenet.com/script/main/art.asp?articlekey=52061

Comment: I am familiar with stress. I worry a lot more than I should. I have little doubt that stress was part of the reason why I became ill with cancer. I know that when I worry, I can feel my body reacting in many ways, none of them good.

Dr. Hamer, a German oncologist, developed cancer in the late '70s, shortly after his son's untimely death. Theorizing that there could be a connection between the stress of his son's death and his development of cancer, he reviewed his cancer patients' histories. Consistent with his theory, he found that these patients also had experienced an unexpected shock or trauma shortly before their cancer. Then, he reviewed his patients' brain scans and compared them with corresponding medical and psychological records. He also found a clear correlation between shock therapy, specific areas of the brain damaged by certain types of shocks, and the particular organs in which cancer developed.

Based on the review of over forty thousand case studies over a number of years, he concluded that every disease originates from a shock or trauma that catches us unexpectedly. The moment the unexpected conflict occurs, the shock strikes a specific area in the brain, causing a lesion (called Hamer—focus) visible on a brain scan as a set of sharp concentric rings in CT scans. The brain cells that receive the impact send a biochemical signal to the corresponding body cells causing the growth of a tumor, a meltdown of tissue or functional loss, depending on which brain layer receives the shock.

He theorized that specific conflicts are tied to specific areas in the brain because during evolution, brain areas are programmed to respond instantly to conflicts that could threaten survival. For example, let's say that a woman is walking with her child. Suddenly the child runs into the street and is struck by a car. The moment a mother sees her child injured, she suffers a mother-child-worry conflict, and in a split second, a special biological program for this particular type of conflict is switched on.

Comment: Hamer's theory is interesting and provocative, but is not universally accepted by the scientific and medical community at large. However, it serves as an interesting topic to debate while considering whether or not stress contributes to cancer, although it is recognized that there are many other underlying causes for cancer than simply being initiated by stressful events. Hamer's reports raise the possibility that stress may be more important in initiating cancer than had been previously thought. What is undoubtedly for certain is that stress can have adverse effects on the immune system that could affect the accelerated growth of cancer cells. Continued stress from unresolved traumatic events *must* inhibit your body's ability to fight cancer.

Comment: I believe your mind can take you in either direction of health. You can make yourself sick with your mind, you also can make yourself better.

The placebo effect is the measurable, observable, or felt improvement in health or behavior not attributable to a medication or treatment that has been administered.

http://www.skepdic.com/placebo.html

"The physician's belief in the treatment and the patient's faith in the physician exert a mutually reinforcing effect; the result is a powerful remedy that is almost guaranteed to produce an improvement and sometimes a cure."

Follies and Fallacies in Medicine, p. 13 Peter Skrabanek and James McCormick.

Factors influencing of the placebo effect include the following:

Placebo Characteristics: If the pill looks genuine, any person taking it is more likely to believe that it contains medicine. Research shows that larger-sized pills suggest a stronger dose than smaller pills, or taking two pills appears to be more potent than swallowing just one. Generally, patients sense that injections have a more powerful effect than pills.

Attitude: If the person expects the treatment to work, the chances of a placebo effect are higher. Some studies show that the placebo effect may still take place even if the person is skeptical of success. The power of suggestion may be at work here.

Doctor-Patient Relationship: If the person trusts his/her health care practitioner, he/she is more likely to believe that the placebo will work.

In addition, three other factors have been proposed to explain placebo-evoked improvement:

i)   release of endorphins in response to the placebo stimulus (the "opioid model");

ii) a learned response to medical intervention (the "conditioning model"); and

iii) a more consciously mediated response (the "meaning" or expectancy model).

Hróbjartsson A. The uncontrollable placebo effect. Eur J Clin Pharmacol, 1996; 50: 345-348.

How Placebos Actually May Work

The underlying physiological mechanisms for the placebo effect are unclear. Some of the theories that have been postulated include:

Self-limiting disorders. Many conditions, such as the common cold, are self-limiting. They will resolve by themselves with or without placebos or drugs; hence, the end of symptoms is merely coincidence.

Remission. The symptoms of some disorders, such as multiple sclerosis and lupus tend to wax and wane. Hence a remission during a course of a placebo treatment may be pure coincidence and unrelated to the placebo treatment.

A change in behavior. The placebo may increase a person's motivation to take better care of his/herself, for example by changing to an improved diet, getting more exercise, or getting more rest, all of which, in turn, may be responsible for the easing of their symptoms.

Altered perception. A person's interpretation of his/her symptoms may change with the expectation of feeling better. For example, a sharp pain may be reinterpreted as an uncomfortable tingling.

Reduced anxiety. Simply by taking the placebo and expecting to feel better, may, in fact, soothe the autonomic nervous system, thereby reducing the levels of stress chemicals, such as adrenaline.

Brain chemicals. Placebos may trigger the release of the body's own natural painkillers, the brain chemicals (neurotransmitters) known as endorphins. The permeability of the blood brain barrier the permeability of the blood brain barrier

Altered brain state. Research indicates that the brain responds to an imagined scene in much the same way as it responds to an actual visualized scene. A placebo may help the brain to remember a time before the onset of symptoms, and then bring about physiological change. This theory is called *'remembered wellness'*.

*http://www.betterhealth.vic.gov.au/bhcv2/bhcArticles.nsf/pages/
Placebo_effect?OpenDocument*

> **Comment:** If you watch "The Secret" you will see a story about a woman who reversed cancer just by watching funny movies all day and believing she was getting better. I would like to remind you that "your mind controls you body". If you are dealing with cancer, you should be aware of your state of mind. A placebo does not have to be a pill.

The placebo effect, also known as nonspecific effects or the subject-expectancy effect, is the phenomenon that a patient's symptoms can be alleviated by an otherwise ineffective treatment simply because the patient expects or believes that it will work.

http://www.sciencedaily.com/articles/p/placebo_effect.htm

> **Comment:** So long story short, your state of mind directly affects your physical being. Live life, think positive and be happy. Your mind controls your body. Being in a stressed out state of mind for prolonged periods of time will have numerous negative effects on your body. Conversely, being happy and relaxed all the time will allow your body to function at its best. There are many ways to adjust to a positive mind state, for example, with yoga, tai chi, the Sedona method, meditation, paraliminals (my number 1 choice) and many more. Whichever you choose, just remember that stress literally destroys your body. As is it not possible to destroy your body and be healthy at the same time, you need to find a way to control your moments of stress.

CHAPTER 25

How Magnetism Affects Your Body

Comment: Everything spins. The sun, the moon, the planets and the stars all revolve. Magnetism is a catalyst for chemical reactions. (How disrupting the magnetism in your body with electromagnetic forces can make you weaker and eventually sick will be discussed in the next chapter). It is recognized that all living cells are electromagnetic by nature. There are only two natural sources of magnetism available to you, your brain and the Earth. About eighty percent of the human brain is composed of astrocyte cells. These cells have the capacity to generate electricity and produce a pulsed, electromagnetic field with efficiency. The Earth provides a supportive, steady state magnetic field, which your body draws on to enhance molecular reactions. These two magnetic fields work together to accomplish magnetic resonance, which dramatically enhances the chemical reactions of the body.[1]

Magnetic Resonance: Magnetic resonance occurs when the brain's pulsed magnetic frequency matches the frequencies of various tissues and organs.[1] This is accomplished in ninety to one minute cycles, mostly while we sleep. Resonance will usually maintain a given frequency for a few seconds to a few minutes. This range depends on the urgency and degree of repair or restoration needed. Magnetic resonance is desirable because it helps repair damage done to cells, helps makes enzymes and enhances immunity.[1-2]

Why do we need to augment naturally occurring magnetism? There are two major factors adversely affecting magnetic resonance.

First, a gradual cyclic decline in our geomagnetic field will leave the atoms of our bodies in a lower energy state, making it more difficult for magnetic resonance to occur.[3] It is estimated that we have lost about 80% of our magnetic field in the last four thousand years.[3-6]

Second, because of the ever developing technological age, the external electromagnetic frequencies to which your body is exposed are higher and stronger than ever before (see chapter on EMFs). As a result, these frequencies override the vital brain function of magnetic resonance with your organs and tissues.[7] As a result, this external interference leaves you fatigued, and over an extended period, can contribute to the development of chronic ailments. This development is due, in part, to a lack of restorative resonance.[7]

1. Becker RO MD, Cross Currents, pp. 234-243
2. Lefebyer M, Wiesendanger M, Cherlin D, Blackinton D, Mehta S. Modulation of Lymphocyte Function in Low Frequency Electric and Magnetic Environments. FASEB, 1992; Abstract #2433
3. Cox, A. Magnetic Field Reversals, Scientific American, Feb 1967; pp. 44-54
4. Gubbins D, Bloxhan J. The Secular Variation of the Earth's Magnetic Field, NATURE, 1985; 317.
5. Gubbins D, Bloxhan J. Scientific American, Dec 1989, pp. 71-75.
6. Velikovsky I. Earth in Upheaval, p. 146.
7. Becker RO, MD. Cross Currents, pp. 218-228.

http://www.magneticosleep.com/magnetism/theory/

Magnetism and Your Body

Magnetism can affect your body in two ways. The first is the Earth-type (or unidirectional) field response. But to properly understand how magnetism helps us, let us go back a step. Atoms make up your body. Atoms are composed of even smaller particles, the largest of which are neutrons, protons, and electrons (Figure. 1).

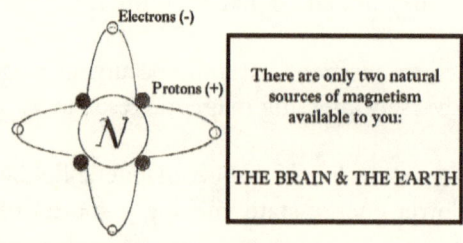

Electrons (-)

Protons (+)

N

There are only two natural sources of magnetism available to you:

THE BRAIN & THE EARTH

If a magnetic field in which an atom exists is increased, the velocity of the electrons and protons will increase or decrease depending on the direction of the magnetic field and the orbits of the particles (Figure 2).[8] The outermost unpaired (valence) electrons are the ones that are shared to make up molecules. These molecules then join to make up the cells that constitute your body.

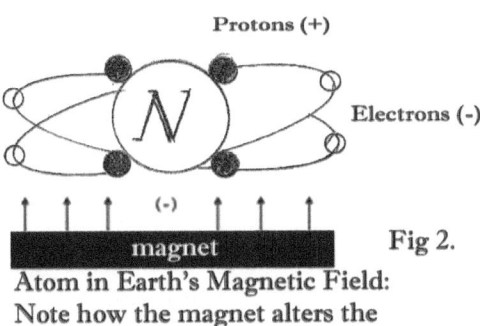

Fig 2.

Atom in Earth's Magnetic Field:
Note how the magnet alters the
electron's orbit.

How Magnetism Affects Atoms

When a magnetic field passes through atoms in the correct direction, it increases their velocity and energy state, which, in turn, enhances the sharing of electrons. The increase of precession or wobble activity in some electrons (depending on the relationship of their orbits to the magnetic field direction) also contributes to this effect. This increased action is a catalyst for chemical reactions in the body. This may remind you fondly or otherwise of high school chemistry experiments, where you heat a solution of two elements to form a new compound. In this sharing of electrons, heat is the catalyst or energy that makes the elements share their electrons.

8. Kip. Fundamentals of Electricity and Magnetism, 1969, pp. 354-357

http://www.magneticosleep.com/magnetism/science-behind-success

> **Comment:** The magnetism in your body is a catalyst for chemical reactions. Magnetism also influences the velocity and energy state of electrons, which are the key difference between free radicals and antioxidants, which, in turn, is a key difference between being healthy and having cancer. There are only a few things you can do to increase the magnetism in your body

properly, such as magnetic bracelets and mattresses. However, one should do his/her homework before making a purchase as there are many scams and ill-informed people selling weak magnets or systems that would incur both negative and positive forces to be applied simultaneously to your body, which is obviously counterproductive. One way to avoid disrupting the magnetic balance in your body would be to remove the inverse of magnetism, which is *"electromagnetic force"*.

CHAPTER 26

Electromagnetic Forces Cause Cancer

Comment: When my cell phone rings near the computer, the computer makes a loud buzz noise. If my cell phone can disrupt the computer signal, I suspect that it also can cause a disruption to my body's electrical impulses as well! In order to understand how electromagnetic forces cause cancer, one needs to first understand electromagnetic forces.

Electromagnetic fields (EMFs) are created by electric power charges. There are two types of fields, electric fields, which result from the strength (voltage) of the charge, and magnetic fields, which result from the motion (amperage) of the charge.

http://www.greenbuilder.com/sourcebook/Emf.html#Define

Comment: Our bodies are made up of all kinds of electrical charges. Disrupting them unquestionably causes problems. Anything that confuses or weakens the cells has the potential to cause a mutation, thus promoting cancer.

According to the National Institute of Environmental Health Sciences, Electric and magnetic fields (EMFs) are invisible lines of force associated with the production, transmission, and use of electric power such as those associated with high-voltage transmission lines, secondary power lines, and home wiring and lighting. Electric and magnetic fields also arise from the motors and heating coils found in electronic equipment and appliances.

Because the use of electric power is so widespread, humans are constantly exposed to electric and magnetic fields. Studies conducted in the 1980s showed a link between magnetic field strength and the risk of childhood leukemia. After reviewing more than two decades of research in this area, NIEHS scientists concluded that the overall pattern of results suggests a weak association between increasing exposure to EMFs and an increased risk of childhood leukemia. The few studies that have been conducted on adult exposures show no evidence of a link between residential EMF exposure and adult cancers, including leukemia, brain cancer, and breast cancer. Based on these reviews, the NIEHS recommends continued education on practical ways of reducing exposures to EMFs.

http://www.niehs.nih.gov/health/topics/agents/emf/

> **Comment:** Studies showed a link between EMFs and childhood leukemia. NIEHS scientists conclude a "weak association" between increased exposure to EMFs and risk of leukemia. But an association was acknowledged nonetheless. Few studies conducted show no evidence of a link, yet experts recommend "continued education on practical ways of reducing exposures to EMFs."

In November 1989, the Department of Energy reported that "It has now become generally accepted that there are, indeed, biological effects due to field exposure."

Here's a funny clip from a government website, "Studies have shown that some workers exposed to high magnetic fields have increased cancer rates. But such associations do not necessarily indicate that EMF exposures cause cancer (any more than the springtime association of robins and daffodils shows that one causes the other). Scientists have looked carefully at all the EMF evidence, but they disagree about the health effects of EMFs except to say that better information is needed."

http://www.cdc.gov/niosh/emf2.html/

> **Comment:** So they did a study, found "increased rates of cancer", but supposedly "experts in the field" say "better information" is needed? This is consistent with the previous article which says that there is "no evidence of a link", but still recommend "reducing exposure to EMFs". The following is what the Environment Protection Agency (EPA) had to say on this.

By 1990, over one hundred studies had been conducted worldwide. Of these, at least two dozen epidemiological studies on humans indicated a link between EMFs and serious health problems. In response to public pressure, EPA began reviewing and evaluating the available literature.

In a draft report issued in March 1990, the EPA recommended that EMFs be classified as a class B carcinogen because it was a "probable" human carcinogen, thus joining the ranks of such agents as formaldehyde, DDT, dioxins and PCBs. After the EPA draft report was released, utility, military and computer lobbyists came down hard on the EPA. As a result, the EPA's final report did NOT classify EMFs as a class B carcinogen. Rather, the EPA added the following explanation, "At this time such a characterization regarding the link between cancer and exposure to EMFs is not appropriate because the basic nature of the interaction between EMFs and biological processes leading to cancer is not understood."

Curiously, this rather unusual logic appears on the same page as the following: "In conclusion, several studies showing that leukemia, lymphoma and cancer of the nervous system in children exposed to EMFs, supported by similar findings in adults in several occupational studies also involving electrical power frequency exposures, show a consistent pattern of response, suggesting a causal link."

When questioned about the contradictory nature of these statements, the EPA responded that it was "not appropriate" to use the "probable carcinogen" label until it could demonstrate how EMFs caused cancer and exactly how much EMF is harmful.

This explanation does not satisfy many critics who claim that the EPA's upper management was influenced by political and economic considerations exerted by utility, computer and military lobbyists.

An enormous amount of electricity is created at power-generating stations and sent across the country through wires that carry high voltages. All power lines radiate electromagnetic fields. The question is, to what intensity are the power lines radiating EMFs near YOUR home? The amount of EMFs coming from a power line depends on its particular configuration. Power companies know which power line configurations are best for reducing EMFs, but most do not feel the evidence supports costly changes to the way they deliver electricity.

Moreover, substations each of which is a composite of circuit breakers, disconnecting switches and transformers, substations have been blamed for causing cancer clusters in adjacent communities. Paul Brodeur wrote about several such cancer clusters in the July 9, 1990 issue of the *New Yorker Magazine*.

A key component of a utility's electrical distribution network also depends upon numerous small transformers mounted on power poles. A transformer looks like a small metal trash can, usually cylindrical. Even when the electrical service is underground, you will often see a metal box (usually square) located on the ground near the street. (Many people do not realize that when they see a transformer, the power line feeding the transformer is 4,000 to 13,800 volts.) The transformers reduce the voltage to the 120/240 volts needed by nearby homes. Since these transformers can be seen in almost every neighborhood, they are a source of concern. EMFs around each transformer can be quite high, but due to its small structure, the field strength diminishes rapidly with distance, as it does from any point source. For this reason, having a transformer located near your home is usually not a major source of concern although just to make sure, everyone should measure the field strength around it.

Home wiring also plays a role in EMF generation. If your home has high EMF readings, it is important to determine the sources of the EMF so that remedial action can be taken, if possible. Many times, a particular room will have a higher EMF reading than other rooms. Check to see if the electricity is coming into the house on the wall outside that room. When this is the case, it is usually a good idea to block off that room and only use it for storage purposes. Sometimes, the source of a high magnetic field is due to incorrect wiring. If you suspect that your home is wired improperly, obtain the services of a licensed electrician. Warning: Do not touch electric wires, even if you think the current is turned off. If you need to disconnect electrical circuits to determine the source of magnetic fields, you should call a licensed electrician.

Computers are a complicated subject. It should be recognized that EMFs radiate from all sides of a computer. Thus, you not only should be concerned about sitting in front of the monitor, but also if you are sitting near a computer or if a computer is operating in a nearby room.

The Swedish safety standard, effective in 1990, specifies that computers should only have a maximum of 0.25 mG at 50 cm from the display. Many US-manufactured computers, however, have EMFs of 5 to100 mG at this distance. And screens placed over monitors do NOT block EMFs, not even a lead screen will block ELF and VLF magnetic fields.

Space does not permit a more thorough discussion of computers. If you use a computer, it is important that you measure your EMF exposure with a gauss meter and review the literature concerning the health impacts of computer use.

Fluorescent lights produce more EMFs than incandescent bulbs. A typical fluorescent lamp in an office ceiling has readings of 160 to 200 mG one inch away.

Microwave Ovens and Radar in military installations and airports emit two types of radiation, microwave and ELF. Microwaves are measured in milliwatt per centimeter squared (mW/cm^2). As of January 1993, the US safety limit for microwave exposure has been 1 mW/cm^2, down from a previously acceptable level of 10 mW/cm^2. In contrast, the Russian safety limit is 0.01 mW/cm^2. All microwave ovens leak and exceed the Russian safety limit. In addition, recent Russian studies have shown that normal microwave cooking converts food protein molecules into carcinogenic substances.

When measuring microwaves from military and airport radar sources, 100% accurate readings can only be found with extremely expensive digital peak-hold meters. Why? Because analog devices begin to drop their reading immediately after the radar sweep passes. Thus, while an analog meter can show whether or not you are being exposed to radar EMFs, analog meters do not show your true exposure. Although thousands of dollars to purchase, digital-hold meters capable of accurately detecting radar EMFs can be rented for several hundred to over a thousand dollars per month.

Telephones and answering machines can emit surprisingly strong EMFs, especially from the handset. This is a problem because we hold the telephone so close to our head. Place the gauss meter right against the earpiece and the mouthpiece before buying a phone. Some brands emit no measurable fields, and others emit strong fields that travel several inches, namely, right into your brain. Answering machines, particularly those with adapter plugs (minitransformers), emit high levels of EMFs.

http://www.mercola.com/article/emf/emf_dangers.htm

> **Comment:** If magnetism is good, then EMFs are bad. Removing them is just one more piece of the equation that is good health.

CHAPTER 27

Why Radio and Chemotherapy Are Bad

Comment: There is no doubt that chemotherapy slows tumor growth. However, it does so by killing bad cells and, unfortunately, good ones as well. These good cells include your NK and T cells, important parts of your immune system. How is a body supposed to fight the last few cancer cells that chemotherapy cannot kill with a weak immune system? Western medicine does not address this immune deficiency while going through chemotherapy. I suggest this is one of the reasons why so many patients relapse after five years. Also, chemotherapy does not address the underlying cause of the cancer problem. What caused the tumor in the first place? Was it toxic overload, stress, malnutrition, an acidic pH level, or something else? Does chemotherapy resolve any of those issues? I certainly do not think so.

Chemotherapy purpose and stats are based on a reduction of tumor size and life extension. Long term survival rates are not addressed. You certainly would not prescribe chemotherapy to a healthy person; that would make him/her sick! So why are we prescribing it to people who are already sick to begin with?

Comment: Let us look at the three classes of chemotherapy drugs and the ways in which they damage cells. Yes, that is correct, all three classes of chemotherapy drug are designed to damage cells. The agents either

1. Prevent the copying of cellular components needed to divide
2. Replace or eliminate essential enzymes or nutrients the cells needed to survive, or
3. Trigger cells to self-destruct

*http://www.curesearch.org/for_parents_and_families/intreatment/medical/article.
aspx?stageid=3&topicid=70&articleid=3126*

Ask anyone undergoing chemotherapy and they will tell you that the goal of chemo treatment is to feel as well as possible for as long as possible, not simply to cure the disease, only to destroy or remove the *current* tumor. "If you can shrink the tumor size to 50% or more for 28 days, you have got the FDA's definition of an 'active' drug. That is called a response rate. So you have a response, but when you look to see if there is any life prolongation from taking this treatment what you find is all kinds of hocus pocus and song and dance about the disease free survival, and this and that. In the end there is no proof that chemotherapy in the vast majority of cases actually extends life, and this is the GREAT LIE about chemotherapy, that somehow there is a correlation between shrinking a tumor and extending the life of the patient."

Ralph Moss PhD

> **Comment:** Radiotherapy makes about as much sense as sticking your head in a microwave. Just as I learned from my own experience, removing the tumor is just removing the tumor. Chemotherapy has nothing to do with reversing the causes of the cancer. It will not even break down cancer cells in their entirety. Unfortunately, it has to do with money.

CHAPTER 28

How to Supercharge Your Body

Comment: Even if you understand already how to prevent and reverse cancer, I suggest very strongly that you continue reading because the following information will greatly enhance your understanding of the previous materials provided.

These are some other things that you should know about when preventing and reversing cancer. I'm not suggesting that you do all these things; that would be unbalanced. But you should know about them and how they relate to this "cancer equation". For example, a car is made up of many parts. You do not just change the tires every time you have a problem with your car, even if you could get the best tires in the world. Your body is one whole unit made of many pieces that must work together in order to function properly. No one thing will work for everyone. Balance is the key. You must be aware of your own weaknesses to focus on repairing whatever damage has been done if you wish to reverse or prevent cancer in the long term, whether it be lack of vitamins, toxicity, poor pH levels, etc.

i) Goji Berries or Wolfberry

Comment: Goji berries are known to have over ninety-seven vitamins, minerals and nutrients. The goji bush can survive a twenty degree temperature change in twenty-four hours. This is one hardy plant. It also is one of the only known species of plant to contain the anticancer mineral germanium (see chapter on oxygen). Goji berries contain a master molecule and polysaccharides that can restore and repair damaged DNA, which, in turn, can help prevent and reverse cancer. However, do not eat them before bed, or you will be bouncing off the walls.

http://hubpages.com/hub/Health-Benefits-of-Goji-Berry

Tibetan Medicine: Deep in the valleys of the Himalayas of Tibet and Mongolia, there grows a red berry about the size of a small grape. This berry, known locally as the goji berry, is celebrated by the locals in two weeklong festivals every year. Revered for thousands of years as a great healer, a natural antiaging supplement, and a nutritional staple, the goji berry, along with its juice, is just now sweeping its way into Western consciousness.

http://www.gojijuices.net/gojijuicestory.html

The benefits of goji berries or *Lycium barbarum* have been known in Tibet for at least 1,700 years. Tibetan medicine includes these berries in the treatment of kidney and liver problems. They also are used in Tibet to lower cholesterol, lower blood pressure, and cleanse the blood.

Goji berries have a long history of use in the treatment of eye problems, skin rashes, psoriasis, allergies, insomnia, chronic liver disease, diabetes, and tuberculosis. Goji berries are also used by the people of Tibet to increase longevity and as a general health strengthening tonic.

http://www.timpanogosnursery.com/site/928760/page/417077

Modern science has shown that this bright red berry not only contains extremely high levels of antioxidants, vitamins, and minerals, but also contains many unique phytochemicals, polysaccharides, and complex compounds that scientists are just beginning to understand.

Goji berries contain the following complex compounds:

Betaine, which is used by the liver to produce choline (a compound that calms nervousness), enhances memory, promotes muscle growth, and protects against fatty liver disease. Physalin is active compound against all major types of leukemia. It also has been used as a treatment for hepatitis B.

Solavetivone is a powerful antifungal and antibacterial compound.

Beta-sitoserol is an anti-inflammatory agent. It has been used to treat sexual impotence and prostate enlargement. It also lowers cholesterol.

Cyperone, which is a sesquiterpene, is thought to benefit the heart and blood pressure. It has also been used in the treatment of cervical cancer.

The goji berry is also being called the world's most powerful anti-aging food. It is rated number 1 on the Oxygen Radical Absorbance Capacity scale (ORAC scale), which measures the antioxidant level in foods, a test developed by USDA researchers at Tufts University in Boston.

http://theunicornangel.com/blog/?p=17

Himalayan goji berries contain *polysaccharides*, which strengthen the immune system. Research studies report that a polysaccharide found in the goji fruit is a powerful *secretagogue* or substance that stimulates the secretion of human growth hormone (HGH) by the pituitary gland. As we get older, we produce less and less HGH. Increased levels of HGH contribute to rejuvenation and anti-aging.

http://www.astrologyzine.com/himalayan-goji-berries.shtml

Goji berries are one of the most nutritionally rich foods, containing the carotenoids (beta-carotene, zeaxanthin, lutein, β-crytoxanthin and lycopene), at least six vitamins (C, B1, B2, B3, B6, and E) over thirty essential and trace elements (polyphenolic antioxidants) and nineteen amino acids.

Macronutrients in Goji

Goji contains significant percentages of a day`s macronutrient needs, carbohydrates, protein, fat and dietary fiber. About 68% of a goji berry exists as a carbohydrate, 12% as protein, 10% fiber and 10% fat, with a total caloric value of 370 for a 100 gram serving.

The seeds of the goji berry contain polyunsaturated fats such as linoleic (omega-6) and linolenic (omega-3) acids.

Micronutrients in Goji

Goji's diversity and high concentration of micronutrients brand it as an exceptional health food.

Calcium is the primary constituent of teeth and bones, calcium also has a diverse role in soft tissues where it is involved in cardiac, neuromuscular, enzymatic, hormonal, and transport mechanisms across cell membranes. Goji berries contain 112 mg per 100 gram serving, providing about 8-10% of the Recommended Daily Intake (RDI).

Potassium is an essential electrolyte and enzyme cofactor, dietary potassium can lower high blood pressure. Giving about 24% of the RDI (1,132mg/100 grams), goji berries are an excellent source.

Iron is an oxygen carrier on hemoglobin, iron also is a cofactor for enzymes involved in numerous metabolic reactions. Goji berry delivers 100% of RDI at 9 mg/100 grams and is regarded as one of the best sources of iron.

Zinc is essential for making proteins, DNA, and the functions of over 100 enzymes. Zinc is involved in critical cell activities such as membrane transport and repair and growth. Zinc in goji berries has a high content at 20% RDI.

Selenium, sometimes called the *antioxidant mineral,* is often included in supplements. Selenium has unusually high concentration in goji berries (50 micrograms/100 grams) at nearly 100% RDI.

Riboflavin (B_2) is an essential vitamin supporting energy metabolism. Riboflavin is needed for synthesizing other vitamins and enzymes. A daily serving of 100 grams provides the complete RDI (1.3mg).

Vitamin C is a universal antioxidant vitamin protecting other antioxidant molecules from free radical damage. The content of vitamin C in dried berries ranges from 29mg to 148mg/100 grams. Even at the lower estimate, 35% of RDI is still provided. Vitamin C content of fresh berries is much higher and provides the full RDI.

Phytochemicals in Goji

Goji berries contain dozens of phytochemicals whose properties are under scientific study. Five of these are of particular interest:

i) Beta-carotene, which is a carotenoid pigment in orange-red foods like goji, pumpkins, carrots and salmon. Beta-carotene is important for synthesis of vitamin A, a fat-soluble nutrient and antioxidant essential for normal growth, vision, cell structure, bones and teeth, and healthy skin. The beta-carotene content in goji berries per unit weight (7 mg/100 grams), which is among the highest for edible plants.

ii) Goji berries are also rich in zeaxanthin, another carotenoid that is important as a retinal antioxidant and pigment filter of ultraviolet light. Goji berries contain 162 mg/100 grams.

iii) Lycopene, unknown previously as a constituent of berry fruit, is found in goji berries in a concentration of 1.4 mg/100 grams (contracted assay, UBE Analytical Labs). Lycopene acts as an antioxidant role and possible cancer-inhibiting agent in microgram amounts in the blood; this is a potentially important discovery that merits further research.

iv) Polysaccharides are long-chain sugar molecules, characteristic of many herbal medicines like mushrooms and roots. Polysaccharides are a signature constituent of goji berries, making up 31% of pulp weight in premium quality goji berries. Polysaccharides are a primary source of fermentable dietary fiber in the intestinal system. Upon colonic metabolism, fermentable or "soluble fibers" yield short-chain fatty acids, which are valuable for health of the colonic mucosal lining, enhance mineral uptake, stabilize blood glucose levels, lower pH and reduce colon cancer risk, and stimulate the immune system. Polysaccharides also display antioxidant activity.

v) Phenolics, also called phenols or polyphenols, are a group of phytochemicals numbers in the thousands of individual chemicals existing across the plant kingdom, mainly as protective astringents or pigments that give bright colors to plants like the ripe red goji berry. Phenolic pigments have the metabolic property of high antioxidant capability transferable to animals by eating the plant. New assays have demonstrated the presence in goji berries of phenolics such as ellagic acid (86 mg/100 grams) and p-coumaric acid, with a total phenolics content of 1,309 mg/100 grams, one of the highest values for any plant food yet tested.

http://www.saskgojipower.ca/gpage.html

Goji stimulates the release by the pituitary gland of HGH (human growth hormone), the youth hormone. The benefits of HGH are extensive and include reduction of body fat, better sleep, improved memory, accelerated healing, restored libido, and a more youthful appearance.

http://www.greenwoodhealth.net/np/ssf/goji.htm

Goji is one of the only plant species on earth that contains the anticancer mineral germanium (see chapter on oxygen). Its antioxidants and unique polysaccharides can halt the genetic mutations that can lead to cancer. Some scientists believe that goji may be an especially good supplement to prevent liver cancer because it exerts liver protection and anticancer effects at the same time. This is important, as the liver is the body's primary detoxifying organ.

http://www.bilbridge.com/BILAdvertising/images/38%20Reasons%20for%20 Drinking%20Goji%20Juice.pdf

Some of the polysaccharides that can be found in goji berries are actually unique to the fruit. All twenty-two of these polysaccharides bring unique benefits for the health of an individual.

Research has also shown that goji berries can now be regarded as a cure-all. Studies in such esteemed journals like the *Journal of EthnoPharmacology, American Journal of Chinese Medicine, Chinese Journal of Pharmacology* and *Toxicology* all praise the effects that goji berries can bring.

http://www.gojifacts.org/goji-juice-benefits-and-goji-research/Goji-Juice- Research-Oh-What-a-Tiny-Fruit-Can-Do.php

Goji Berries and Oxygen Radical Absorbance Capacity

ORAC is the standard test adopted by the US Department of Agriculture, developed by scientist at Tufts University to measure the potency of antioxidants in food. The test was developed by Dr. Guohua Cao, a physician and chemist who worked at the National Institute on Aging in Baltimore, Maryland. The ORAC test, though not the be all and end all of antioxidant testing, gives a good idea of the free-radical-destroying potential of a given food. It does this by measuring the time an antioxidant takes to react as well as the capacity of antioxidants within the sample food. It combines these elements into one measurement that is commonly expressed in terms of a 100 gram sample.

It has been suggested that humans should consume about 5,000 ORAC units a day for maximum benefits. Unfortunately, most people do not eat nearly enough vegetables and fruit, or the right type of vegetables and fruit, to achieve this. For example, to get your daily ORAC dose from apples, you would need to eat 2,294 grams of apple (or about twenty-two apples). However, as you can see from the chart below chart, eating just 20 grams of goji berries will cover you.

It is important to remember, however, that there is a lot more to measuring a food's antioxidant capacity than ORAC. Since different antioxidants have different effects, it is still important to eat a variety of foods (including apples) with high antioxidant levels. For example, although strawberries have a higher ORAC score than spinach, spinach has been shown to be more effective than strawberries in boosting blood antioxidant scores. So although eating a large amount of antioxidants is always a plus, it is important to eat a variety of healthy foods, not only for their antioxidant levels, but for their other nutritional properties as well.

Fruits	ORAC Score (/100 grams)	Grams Needed to Reach DRI
Goji Berries	25,300-30,300	20
Mangosteen	20,000	
Acai	18,400	
Black Raspberries	5,100-7,700	65
Prunes	5,770	87
Bilberry	4,460	112
Boysenberry	3,500	
Pomegranates	3,307-10,500	151
Raisins	2,830	177
Plums	2,800	
Blueberries	2,400	208
Red Raspberries	2,400	208
Blackberries	2,036-5,100	246
Noni	1,706	
Strawberries	1,540-2,600	325
Noni Fruit	1,506	332
Plums	949	527
Oranges	750-2,400	667
Cherries	670-2,100	746
Red Grapes	739	677
Pink Grapefruit	495	1,010
White Grapefruit	460	1,087
Apples	218-1,400	2,294
Banana	210	2,381
Pears	134	3,731
Watermelon	100	5,000

Vegetables	ORAC Score (per 100 grams)	Grams Needed to Reach DRI
Artichoke	8,100	
Garlic	1,939	258
Spinach	1,770	282
Steamed Spinach	909	550
Yellow Squash	1,550	435
Brussel Sprouts	980	510
Alfalfa Sprouts	930	538

Broccoli	880	568
Beets	840	595
Avocado	782	639
Red Bell Pepper	710	704
Baked Beans	503	994
Onions	450	1,111
Corn	400	1,250
Frozen Peas	375	1,333
Eggplant	390	1,282
Potato	300	1,667
Sweet Potato	295	1,695
Cabbage	295	1,695
Cauliflower	385	1,299
Carrot	210	2,381
Tomato	195	2,564
Cucumber	60	8,333

Other	ORAC Score (/100 grams)	Grams Needed to Reach DRI
Unprocessed Cocoa Powder	8,260-26,000	
Dark Chocolate	13,120	38.1
Milk Chocolate	6,740	74.2
Walnuts	4,062	
Rooibos Tea (200 ml)	750	133

http://www.chocolate-news.org/thumbnails/orac_antioxidant_value_list.JPG

http://thehealthpost.com/wp-content/uploads/2009/03/orac.jpg

http://www.allchocolate.com/images/Content%20Charts/4.2.1-ORAC_BarChart.gif

> **Comment:** There seems to be a misconception that there is no clinical evidence on the content and powers of the goji berry and the noni fruit. This website (*www.PubMed.Gov*) or (*http://www.ncbi. nlm.nih.gov/sites/entrez*) has over 100 published clinical trials; just type in the plant species name.

ii) Noni Fruit

> **Comment:** *Morinda citrifolia* is a tree that produces a lumpy, waxy-looking fruit about the size of a potato that ranges in color as it ripens from green, to yellow, to almost white when it is ripe. Noni trees grow mostly in rich volcanic soil in locations with vast amounts of sun. Growing over sixty feet high, they are

147

the only tree to bear fruit 365 days a year. Containing over 140 vitamins, minerals, and nutrients, noni juice is great for replacing a multivitamin and for the immune system. I supposed this would explain why it was included in the U.S. World War II Military Field Handbook for Survival.

Noni Directly Affects the Body's Cells

Noni literally has the ability to open up the cell wall, allowing more nutrients, like various vitamins and minerals, to be absorbed into our cells and more waste material to be removed from weak or damaged cells. It increases cellular activity, nutritional intake of vitamins, minerals and other nutrients, waste removal, and overall cellular health. This is another reason why noni juice, as a nutritional supplement seems to help such a myriad of health complaints in all body types. This is a nutritional supplement that affects the body in a positive way on a cellular level no matter what the health issue or complaint may be.

http://www.healthy-vitamins-rx.com/html/noni_-cells.html

One proposed explanation is related to the mystical alkaloid called "*xeronine*", that is proposed to work at the cellular level to modify and strengthen the structure of proteins in our cells.

Another theory is that noni contains a selection of polysaccharide compounds that are able to stimulate and enhance the body's own natural immune system.

Noni has also been shown to encourage the body to produce nitric oxide that may aid in fighting tumors and viral, bacterial, and parasitic infections. The proteins in your body's cells are made up of organic material. Some of these hold you together like your skin, hair, and bones. Others at the cellular level are the functional proteins that help cells do work such as enzymes, hormones, antibodies, and cell membrane receptors. Xeronine is believed to have profound effects on the functional proteins in your body that may explain the broad influence noni has on the different systems in your body.

http://www.trunoni.com/8_how_noni_juice_works.htm

Digestive Stimulant: Noni juice has traditionally been used as a laxative.

Antioxidants: Research has shown that noni juice exhibits better antioxidant activity than grape seed extract and pycnogenol, another type of antioxidant.

Analgesic: The noni tree is also known as the "painkiller and headache tree". Noni has been found to be 75% as effective as morphine sulphate in relieving pain without the toxic side effects.

Antibacterial, antifungal and antiparasitic: With the presence of active compounds like anthraquinones, scopoletin, and terpenes, noni is effective against bacteria and fungus.

Anti-inflammatory: Noni juice has shown similar results to the newer over-the-counter anti-inflammatory drugs, called nonsteroidal anti-inflammatory drugs (NSAIDs) such as aspirin and tylenol.

Antitumor/anticancerous: Noni juice contains noni-ppt, which has shown antitumor activity.

http://www.healingnoni.com/noni-juice-benefits.html

Comment: Noni has also been used for the following:

Diarrhea
Intestinal parasites
Indigestion
Stomach ulcers
Arthritis
Sprains
Diabetes
Headaches
Tumors
Fevers
Eye infections
Inflamed gums
Sore throat with cough
Toothaches
Coughs
Tuberculosis
Asthma
Respiratory afflictions
Menstrual cramps

Prostate complaints

> **Comment:** Bad drugs are knowingly put on the shelves and then taken off quietly two years later. Yet they spend all day warning you to be wary of "supposedly" unsubstantiated claims on fruit juice. From a certain standpoint, cannot healthy food be considered the biggest competitor for pharmaceutical companies?

iii) Acai Berry

> **Comment:** Acai berries are great for digestion because they increase your metabolism and have lots of essential fatty acids.

Acai or *Euterpe oleracea* (pronounced AH-sci-EE) juice is the newest of these four juices to be introduced. It comes from the Brazilian rainforest, where it kept people alive during times of famine. It is one of the few plant foods that are high in a complete source of protein. It is also rich in essential fatty acids like the omega-3, 6, and 9. It is known as the "beauty berry" and used for premature aging and for beautiful hair, skin and nails. It is also full of fiber and good for digestion. Acai also contains lots of antioxidants and many other beneficial compounds. It has prized by Brazilian natives for its ability to provide energy and a high nutritional content and increase strength. It was traditionally grinded to a pulp and eaten for breakfast or perhaps as an energizing snack later in the day.

The acai berry has twice the level of antioxidants of blueberries and very high levels of omega fatty acids. It is also high in proteins and is a complete source of amino acids, including the essential fatty acids that our body is unable to manufacture. It is a healthy source of fiber and can hence help maintain a healthy digestive system. In addition, it contains phytosterols, which are compounds of plant membranes that can provide many benefits.

Acai has a taste that is described by some as a mix between chocolate and berries. It is deep purple in color and very rich in the class of antioxidants known as anthocyanins. These, like other antioxidants, fight free radicals and help to combat premature aging and even help prevent serious diseases caused or exacerbated by free radical damage like heart disease and cancer.

Other Benefits of Acai Juice as Nutritional Supplement

Supports healthy libido

Supports liver function
Healthy hair, skin and nails
Cleansing and detoxification
Anti-aging and longevity
Mental clarity, good focus and a positive mood

http://www.healthy-vitamins-rx.com/html/acai-juice.html

The proanthocyanidine contents in acai berries are ten to thirty times the anthocyanins (these are the purple colored antioxidants) of red wine per volume.

Rogez H. Acai: Preparo, ComposiÁao, e Melhormento da ConveraÁao. Belem: EDUFPA; 2000.

Nutritional Chemistry of Acai

Polyphenols: 16 (14-212 mg/L)
Anthocyanidins: Thirty times the amount in red wine.
Phytosterols monounsaturated (healthy) fats (fatty acid ratio resembling olive oil): including essential omega fatty acids and Oleic (omega-9)
Polyunsaturated fatty acids: Linoleic (omega-6)
Alpha-tocopherol: natural vitamin E
Trace minerals: copper, iron, calcium, cobalt, chromium and manganese
Dietary Fiber: 7 grams/100 grams
Protein: amino acid profile similar to low glycemic index

Content per 100 grams of Acai:
Acid: 0.13%
Brix: 45.90 g
Protein: 6%
Fiber: 16.9g
Niacin: 0.40mg
Phosphorous: 58mg
Iron: 11.8mg
Vitamin B1: 0.36mg
Vitamin B2: 0.01mg
Calcium: 9mg
Vitamin C: 9mg
pH: 5.21
Calories: 247

Omega fatty acids (omega-9, omega-6 and omega-3). These mono-saturated essential fatty acids help lower low density lipoprotein (LDL), the harmful cholesterol, while maintaining high density lipoproteins (HDL0, the beneficial cholesterol. This unique ratio resembles the same combination as olive oil. Omega fatty acids combat heart disease by increasing healthy cell development. Omega fatty acids are essential for healthy nervous system development and regeneration. They help rapidly repair and rejuvenate muscles after intense exercise.

http://www.acaiberryjuice.org/

Acai has fatty acid content similar to that of olive oil and is rich in monounsaturated oleic acid. This oleic acid helps the penetration of the cell membrane by omega-3 fish oils with which it is possible to make cell membranes supple. A supple cell membrane helps in the efficient functioning of hormones, neurotransmitters, and insulin receptors. The antioxidant properties of acai also helps in the prevention of heart and vascular disease. This is why acai is used extensively in the production of dietary supplements and other products.

The antioxidants in acai are known to improve eyesight and to fight and regulate the cholesterol levels in the body. Acai is also important in maintaining the cardiovascular system to promote better blood circulation. These antioxidants are effective in removing free radicals from the body and improving cell growth. With the damaging effects of free radicals removed from the body, the acai berry boosts the body's immune system and provides it with protection from free radical damage.

http://acaiproductsplus.com/

> **Comment:** I cannot believe there are so many major juice companies that use the whole berry inclusive to the seed in their juice. The nutritional information is based on the skin and pulp, not the seed, which has not been tested for human consumption. My understanding is that in the rainforest where acai comes from they make jewelry out of the seed. They do not eat it. Always check the label. Do not get misled by fancy marketing. Most things that say acai on the label have almost no acai in it. But that being said, for me acai is part of my daily regimen.

iv) Mangosteen

> **Comment:** Mangosteen, sometimes referred to as "the *queen of fruits*" reminds me of an orange. But instead, it has a thick purple

peel with a white instead of orange inside. It is great for the immune system, and it has antioxidant qualities.

A Powerful Whole Food Nutritional Supplement

Most mangosteen (*Garcinia mangostana*) juice comes from places in Southeast Asia like Thailand and Indonesia. It has long been used both as a table fruit and in folk and traditional medicine for inflammatory conditions of the bowel, to help control pain, to disinfect wounds and more. The key active therapeutic ingredients in mangosteen are the phytonutrients called xanthones.

Powerful Natural Anti-inflammatory Xanthones in Mangosteen Juice

These phytonutrients are natural anti-inflammatory agents, and it turns out that the mangosteen fruit and its juice are nature's richest known source of these xanthones, found mostly in its rind. Xanthones have been shown to be cyclooxygenase-1 and-2 (COX-1 and COX-2) inhibitors, which are used in synthetic versions in various pharmaceutical drugs for patients with severe osteoarthritis, rheumatoid arthritis, or other inflammatory conditions. Some of these Rx drugs include Celebrex® and Vioxx®, which have recently been in the media as potentially unsafe drugs.

In addition to helping with pain, reducing inflammation in the body may be critical to lowering the incidence of all sorts of chronic degenerative diseases, like cancer, heart disease, lupus, Crohn's disease, Alzheimers and ulcerative colitis.

Powerful Antioxidants Contained in Mangosteen

These xanthones are also powerful antioxidants, and hence can reduce free radical damage in your body. Free radical damage in your body may manifest itself as premature aging, elevated bad cholesterol (LDL), cell and DNA mutations, cardiovascular disease and more; so if you can reduce any of those, it may be very helpful.

Mangosteen is a Natural Immune Booster

Researchers in Asia have shown that the xanthones in mangosteen are powerful stimulants to the immune system. Current research is showing that xanthones may even be effective against liver, breast and colon cancer, as well as leukemia.

Natural Antibacterial and Antifungal Properties of Mangosteen

As you probably have heard, overuse of antibiotics in many parts of the world has created strains of drug-resistant bacteria. One of these resistant strains is one of the staph bacteria called MRSA. Scientists in experiments have seen strong antibacterial activity against MRSA and other super strains of bacteria. Xanthones also show strong antifungal activity.

Mangosteen Acts as a Natural Anti-histamine

Histamines are released in the body by allergen-sensitive people when they are exposed to an allergen; e.g., pollen, dust, foods, pet dander, and feather pillows. *In vitro*, the xanthones in mangosteen have shown to directly lower histamine release. This means that the xanthones in mangosteen and mangosteen juice may very likely be a great natural support for those with allergies.

Unfortunately, most mangosteen juice sold today is diluted with water and other fruit juices and may not contain very many of these powerful xanthones.

http://www.healthy-vitamins-rx.com/html/mangosteen-juice.html

Mangosteen's Anti-cancer Properties

Researchers have shown that the xanthones compound found in the mangosteen fruit carry the properties of antileukemia, antitumor (shrinks the tumor in the body), antifungal (critical for all cancer patients), antibacterial (protects the DNA), antioxidants, and antiproliferation (kills cancer cells). This is perhaps why the mangosteen is revered as a possible cancer cure.

http://ezinearticles.com/?Mangosteen-and-Cancer&id=408771

http://ezinearticles.com/?expert=Kevin_Stith

> **Comment:** Check out Dr. Templeman and Dr. Morton for more information on mangosteen and cancer. They claim that mangosteen outperforms five of six cancer drugs *in vitro* (in the test tube).

v) Spirulina, Phytoplankton, Chlorella, AFA or Blue-Green Algae

> **Comment:** There is a lot of life in the sea, a lot of vitamins and a lot of minerals. Imagine if the tree in your backyard had roots that reached all across the globe. How many vitamins, minerals, and nutrients would it have access to? If you look at the "amino acid profile chart" for algae, you would think that it had been specifically designed to match the ratio of human amino acids required by the body. Also, I would like to remind you that your DNA is made of amino acids.

AFA happens to have the highest concentration of chlorophyll than any other food in the world. Why is this significant? There is a link between chlorophyll, (the blood of the plant kingdom) and hemoglobin (the blood of the animal kingdom). Chlorophyll is vital for the body's rapid assimilation of amino acids.

In addition to the many benefits of increased oxygen in the body, AFA also possesses specific nutrients, which cross the blood-brain barrier to directly nourish the brain.

http://www.breathing.com/e3live.htm

AFA is a very nutritious whole food containing over sixty-four nutrients that are 97% absorbed by the body. It supplies small amounts of premium quality nutrients generally lacking from our diet—virtually every nutrient—in an energetic form that maximizes their benefits because it is harvested wild and is processed correctly. These algae may be of help with cancer.

AFA contains high amounts of chlorophyll and, therefore, is an excellent detoxifier. Chlorophyll is thought to be especially valuable for dealing with cancer, because its structure is very similar to hemoglobin. Thus, some claim it may help transport oxygen. AFA also is a concentrated green food, and therefore, is very alkalinizing (see chapter on pH).

The basis of life. Billions of years old. Cell biologists say that the enzyme system in the AFA algae is virtually identical to the enzyme system in our cellular mitochondria. The mitochondria is what produces the energy in our cells.

AFA contains a significant amount (about 3 to 5% by weight) of the essential omega-3 fatty acid linolenic acid. The essential fatty acids present in it are remarkably bioavailable and lead to the accumulation in the blood of EPA and DHA, two long chain fatty acids associated with brain function and cardiovascular health. In addition, it leads to a decrease in the blood of the inflammatory fatty acid arachidonic acid.

This data suggests that these blue-green algae are a good dietary supplement to prevent deficiency in omega-3 fatty acids. Our cells need an adequate supply of omega-3 fatty acids to oxygenate properly (see chapter on oxygen). In addition, its has a proven effect at enhancing natural killer cell activity by 40%!

Klamath blue-green algae are the most nutrient dense food on the planet, containing glycoproteins, vitamins, minerals, simple carbohydrates, lipids and biologically active enzymes. Due to the algae's nutritious soft cell wall, these nutrients are readily available to the body. As the body uses only a small amount of energy to convert this "super food" into fuel, consuming Klamath blue-green algae is a fast, efficient and energizing way to improve any diet. The discovery of the incredible food value concentrated in AFA (Aphanizomenon Flos Aquae), an ancient blue-green microalgae, has popularized this nutrient dense whole food that contains more protein, B12, and chlorophyll than any other food source.

http://www.klamathbluegreen.com/information-about-klamath-blue-green-algae/information-about-algae-klamath-lake-blue-green-algae-afa-blue-green-algae-blue-green.html

One thousand times better at getting immune cells where they need to go.

In the largest and most extensive study to date, blue-green algae were shown to stimulate immune cell migration, the process that gets the immune cells to where they need to go.

Research has also shown that AFA contains the polysaccharide responsible for stimulating the immune system. The University of Mississippi in the United States isolated this polysaccharide from AFA and showed that it has the ability to stimulate macrophage activity in the front line of the immune system. This study demonstrated that these polysaccharides are between one hundred to one thousand times more active than polysaccharide preparations that are currently used to treat cancer.

But Campbell pointed out that people think in terms of stimulating the immune system, and we forget that the immune system is by far the main producer of inflammatory mediators and free radicals. Stimulating the immune system also may mean promoting inflammation and enhancing oxidation in the body. AFA does not let that happen.

It is the color in the compound that fights inflammation.

AFA keeps the immune system from being overstimulated to the point where it causes more harm than good, which actually makes it even more effective as an anti-inflammatory.

1. JANA 2000; 2(3): 50-8
2. Planta Medica 2001; 67(8): 737-42
3. Inflamm Res 1998; 47: 36-41
4. Biochem Biophys Res Commun 2000; 277(3): 599-603
5. JANA 2001; 3(4): 24-30

http://www.thehealthierlife.co.uk/natural-health-articles/immunity/blue-green-algae-boost-immune-system-00649.html

> **Comment:** Upper Klamath Lake is the largest freshwater lake in Oregon and one of the largest in the United States.

Algae capitalize on the direct energy of the sun more than any other food. Primitive as they may appear, most are highly efficient photosynthesizers. Algae utilize light energy from the sun (greater than 10% conversion efficiency), carbon dioxide from the air, and hydrogen from the water to synthesize its biochemicals.

Foundation Food

Algae have been eaten in various forms for thousands of years. They are rich in beta-carotene and B-complex, biologically active vitamins, enzymes, chlorophyll, fatty acids, neuropeptide precursors (peptides are joined amino acids), lipids, carbohydrates, minerals, trace minerals, pigments, and other essential growth factors. They contain all eight essential amino acids and both semiessential amino acids. They are a concentrated source of arginine, known to build and tone muscle tissue. Most importantly, the essential amino acid profile of AFA is virtually identical to that required by the human body. No vital amino acid is wasted.

In trying to understand the physiological benefits of blue-green algae, we must also consider the impressive list of sugars it creates: alginics, fucoidins, galactans, agars, laminarins, mannans, ribose, to name only a few (Armstrong F., 1983). The algae use these complex sugars for all its biochemical needs, such as the building, repairing, and replacing of damaged structures.

Research has shown that it is not only what you eat, but what your body absorbs and assimilates that is important. Microalgae, existing at the beginning of the food chain, provide the simplest form of balanced, whole food nutrients. Klamath blue-reen algae have a very nutritious, easily digested, soft cell wall, comprised of a glucolipoprotein complex. This allows rapid absorption of vital nutrients with 95% assimilation, at almost no cost to the body's digestive energy supplies. Most of the nutrients in AFA are active and in forms that are directly useable by the body.

Brain Food

"The greatest value of A.F.A. is not only its nutrient concentration, but its effect on the nervous system, specifically the pituitary, pineal, and hypothalamus. People taking A.F.A. have reported an overall increase in mental alertness, mental stamina, short and long term memory, problem solving, creativity, dream recall, a greater sense of well being and centeredness."

DrGabriel Cousens, MD, author in Body, Mind, Spirit, April 1995

"A tiny protein called substance P is a powerful neurotransmitter. It is composed of arginine, lysine, and proline, all of which are available in AFA. The amazing effect of substance P is that it enhances learning ability and elevates our sense of well being. It does this by stimulating the brain cells to grow more dendritic spines of brain cell "arms" that reach out and communicate with other brain cells."

Algae to the Rescue, Karl J. Abrams

The metabolism of nitrogen directly from the air allows for the biosynthesis of low molecular weight peptide groups. These are precursors of neurotransmitters, which are used by various regions of the brain and body to initiate the secretion of substances (such as hormones) that influence metabolic functions. These precursors have an overall positive effect on the nervous system. The ability of brain neurons to manufacture and utilize neurotransmitters is dependent upon the concentration of amino acids in the bloodstream. Some of AFA's amino acids actually cross the blood-brain barrier in exactly the form they are found in the algae. Few other foods can make this claim.

Complete Protein

Protein is a central part of the body's energy; it provides for the replication and repair of cells, organs, and organ systems. Protein comprises a major portion of the blood and lymph and creates a natural immunity by giving the body a means of recognizing invading foreign cells and viruses.

Most foods contain lipoproteins that the body must convert to glycoproteins before they can be used. Klamath blue-green algae contain both glycoproteins and carbohydrates, so the body has access to these nutrients without using the body's own digestive energy reserves to convert them first. This is why small amounts can have such tremendous effects.

Protein is made up of amino acids, the "building blocks" of the entire body. Eight of the amino acids are considered "essential" because they cannot be produced inside the body; they must be assimilated from the food we eat. Two are considered semiessential because they are necessary for proper growth in children. The other twelve amino acids are produced within the body. Proper quantities of all twenty-two amino acids (a low amount will limit the assimilation of the higher amounts) are required to maintain health in the body, aiding in the construction of new tissue, enzymes, and hormones.

http://www.klamathbluegreen.com/information-about-klamath-blue-green-algae/information-about-algae-klamath-lake-blue-green-algae-afa-blue-green-algae-blue-green.html

Science News

Cancer-inhibiting Compound Found in the Sea

Science Daily (Aug. 10, 2008) University of Florida College of Pharmacy researchers have discovered a marine compound off the coast of Key Largo that inhibits cancer cell growth in laboratory tests, a finding they hope will fuel the development of new drugs to better battle the disease.

An initial set of papers in the Journal of the American Chemical Society also has garnered the attention of other scientists, and the lab is racing to complete additional research. The molecule's natural chemical structure and ability to inhibit cancer cell growth were first described in the *Science Daily* journal in

February and the laboratory synthesis and description of the molecular basis for its anti-cancer activity appeared July 2.

"It is exciting because we have found a compound in nature that may one day surpass a currently marketed drug or could become the structural template for rationally designed drugs with improved selectivity" said Hendrik Luesch, PhD, an assistant professor in UF's department of medicinal chemistry and the study's principal investigator.

Although scientists have been probing the depths of the ocean for marine products since the early 1960s, many pharmaceutical companies lost interest before researchers could deliver useful compounds because natural products were considered too costly and time-consuming to research and develop.

Many common medications, from pain relievers to cholesterol-reducing statins, stem from natural products that grow on the earth, but there is literally an ocean of compounds yet to be discovered in our seas. Only 14 marine natural products developed are in clinical trials today, Luesch said, and one drug recently approved in Europe is the first-ever marine-derived anticancer agent.

"We have only scratched the surface of the chemical diversity in the ocean," Luesch said. "The opportunities for marine drug discovery are spectacular."

University of Florida

http://www.sciencedaily.com/releases/2008/08/080807175446.htm

CHAPTER 29

Acupuncture and Traditional Chinese Medicine

Comment: I had been going to acupuncture twice a week for well over a year. Now I go every two weeks. My most favorite thing about acupuncture is the way the whole body is considered as one piece. There is no doubt to me, that acupuncture was responsible for a large part of my recovery. It appears to be the whole of recovery for some cancer patients. I have met a gentleman whose terminal cancer of the spine was reversed by my very own acupuncture doctor. This is not the only person with whom my acupuncture doctor has achieved this success. With a good doctor, acupuncture is fantastic. I have learned a different perception on health, nutrition, psychology and lifestyle. For me, my acupuncture doctor is family, which is how I am treated when I am there.

The classical Chinese explanation is that channels of energy run in regular patterns through the body and over its surface. These energy channels, called meridians, are like rivers flowing through the body to irrigate and nourish the tissues. An obstruction in the movement of these energy rivers is like a dam that backs up in others.

The meridians can be influenced by needling the acupuncture points; the acupuncture needles unblock the obstructions at the dams and reestablish the regular flow through the meridians. Acupuncture treatments can therefore help the body's internal organs to correct imbalances in their digestion, absorption, and energy production activities, and facilitate the circulation of energy through the meridians.

The modern scientific explanation is that needling the acupuncture points stimulates the nervous system to release chemicals in the muscles, spinal cord, and brain. These chemicals will either change the experience of pain, or they will trigger the release of other chemicals and hormones, which, in turn, influence the body's own internal regulating system.

The improved energy and biochemical balance produced by acupuncture results in stimulating the body's natural healing abilities and in promoting physical and emotional well-being.

http://www.medicalacupuncture.org/acu_info/articles/aboutacupuncture.html

> **Comment:** After studying the cardiovascular system, the lymphatic system and the meridian lines of acupuncture, I have noticed many similarities. The flow of these systems seems to run in parallel with each other. When you get even the smallest sliver, you body sends a signal to your brain. You then get a pain signal and a subconscious repair signal. When you insert an acupuncture needle, the same equation must be occurring.

> **Comment:** In China (where a large part of the world's population and the planets oldest medicinal practices are located), the government pays for a portion of acupuncture and herbal remedies. The Chinese government encourages the use of natural remedies, and I can understand why. During about my tenth visit to my acupuncturist, after the insertion of the needles, I felt like I was being plugged into a car battery. The experience was intense to say the least. Most of the time now, I just feel like I could pick up the back of a car or maybe shoot lightning bolts out of my fingertips. If I can manage financially, I will go for the rest of my life.

> Acupuncture helps facilitate a healthy body, and in a healthy body, cancer cannot survive.

CHAPTER 30

Paraliminals a.k.a. Binaural Beats

Comment: There are many ways to deal with stress. This one is my personal favorite. Your brain tells your body what to do. The brain frequency for most activities and addictions has been figured out. There is a method to encourage your brain to operate at these specific frequencies. With this assistance, it is possible to guide our brain's frequency to do many things like sleep, concentrate or even heal. This is what I like to think of as the background music that plays in your home. It can directly affect your state of mind, which will directly affect your health. There are many different styles of "binaural beats", they each have their appropriate occasions. Each one can affect how you feel inside in a different way, sort of like tuning your brain like a radio. I use binaural beats mostly to keep me calm and to go to sleep at night.

A binaural beat is a frequency that the brain detects.

This is how it works.

If you play a certain frequency in one ear and a different frequency in the other ear, the brain will detect the difference in frequency. Using the example of the theta brainwave, if you play one frequency at 100 hertz in one ear and the other ear receives a frequency of 107 hertz, then the brain will detect a frequency of 7 hertz. When the brain detects the frequency of 7 hertz, its very own brainwave will fall into sync with the 7 hertz frequency, thus, inducing the brain into the theta brainwave state.

http://www.brainwave-entrainment.com/

Comment: Binaural beats deserve a small book onto itself. But here is one example of what it can do for you physically.

Your brain cells reset their sodium and potassium ratios when the brain is in theta state. The sodium and potassium levels are involved in osmosis, which is the chemical process that transports chemicals into and out of your brain cells. After an extended period in the beta state, the ratio between potassium and sodium is out of balance. This is the main cause of what is known as "mental fatigue". A brief period in theta (about five to fifteen minutes) can restore the ratio to normal resulting in mental refreshment.

http://www.web-us.com/thescience.htm#Various%20Uses%20Of%20Audio%20 With%20Embedded%20Binaural%20Beats

> **Comment:** When meditating, some monks hum the sound "*ohm*". I suggest this is a low binaural frequency that helps induce a trance or meditative state.

> **Comment:** The reason that binaural beats are valuable is because with this method, you are able to guide your brain into any state of mind (or frequency) that you choose. There are many free binaural beats you can download off the Internet as well as many CDs that you can buy. I even have nine different applications with binaural beats on my iPhone for Chakra balance, deep sleep, stress relief, learning enhancement, confidence, wake up, theta, delta and meditation, only to name a few. A good set of headphones will enhance the experience.

CHAPTER 31

MGN-3 and AHCC

Comment: This relates to mega-strengthening your immune system. A weak immune system is usually what kills chemotherapy treated-patients and patients with AIDS. Remember your immune system is the last line of defense against cancer. If you have cancer or especially if you are undergoing chemotherapy, I suggest very strongly that you learn more about and consider adding mushrooms or their nutrients to your diet.

Mushroom glycol nutrients (MGN-3) are a combination of natural nontoxic extracts produced by integrating, through hydrolysis, an extract from the outer shell of rice bran with the extracts from three different mushrooms, shiitake (yielding lentinan), kawaratake (yielding krestin) and suehirotake (yielding sizofiran). In Japan, extracts of rice bran have shown strong antiviral effects, and the three mushrooms used herein have become the three leading prescriptions for the treatment of cancer.

MGN-3 specifically increases the population of natural killer (NK) cells and improves NK activity. NK cells are the body's first line of immune response, making up 15% of our white blood cell count. Each NK cell contains some very specific molecular granules, which act as an ammunition of sorts; the NK cell attaches itself to an enemy invader (like a cancer cell) and injects these granules into its interior, which then explode within five minutes, destroying the invader cell completely while the NK cell remains unharmed and free to move on to destroy other enemy cells and viruses. MGN-3 can increase NK activity by as much as 300%, T-cell activity by 200% and B cell activity by 250%.

MGN-3 increases the number of explosive granules in NK cells. The more granules a NK cell carries, the more powerful it is, and the more virus infected cells it can destroy. MGN-3 also works to increase interferon levels, another potent compound produced by the body that both inhibits the replication of viruses and other parasites while increasing NK cell activity.

MGN-3 also increases the formation of tumor necrosis factor (TNF). TNF is a group of proteins that help destroy cancer cells.

MGN-3 has been studied for many years, and has been shown to work effectively against cancers that are unaffected by angiogenesis inhibitors (like shark cartilage), multiple myleloma (e.g., prostate cancers, breast cancers, ovarian cancer) and appears to be able to lessen the side effects of traditional cancer therapies while effectively eradicating precancerous cell populations.

http://www.vaxa.com/ingredients/MGN-3.cfm

BIOBRAN MGN-3, a nontoxic glycol nutritional food supplement (or functional food) made from breaking down rice bran with enzymes from the shitake mushroom, has been clinically proven to help powerfully enhance depleted immune systems. So successful is this unique and patented MGN-3 arabinoxylan supplement at stimulating immune function that Professor M. Ghoneum of Drew University of Medicine and Science stated that "I have been researching immune modulators for over thirty years now, and Biobran MGN-3 is the most powerful immune complex I have ever tested."

There are other health supplements on the market trying to ride on the back of Biobran MGN-3 research, claiming that they are superior. Perhaps they do this because they are not prepared to spend the money on proper clinical research. In contrast, Biobran MGN-3 now has many years of clinical research behind it, including peer-reviewed papers, which is why it continues to be the leading immune modulator recommended by doctors worldwide.

If your health is at stake, reject any immune modulator that relies on marketing rather than science, and choose one with a proven track record, such as Biobran MGN-3, which is manufactured in Japan. It has been used clinically for over ten years and, in this time, has come to be recognized as the world's leading natural immune modulator.

http://www.biobran.org/

> **Comment:** Active hexose correlated compound (AHCC) is very similar to MGN-3 but is derived, using slightly different combination of mushrooms.

The most notable observed effects of AHCC have been seen in enhancing or boosting the immune system to allow other cancer treatments such as radiation or chemotherapy to work more effectively. It has been reported that AHCC increases the strength of the body's natural defense mechanisms by increasing the body's tolerance of other cancer treatments and, therefore, increasing the effectiveness of those treatments.

http://ahcc-nutrients.com/AHCC-Cancer.html

> **Comment:** To learn more about the clinical research on AHCC, visit *http://www.ahccresearch.com/*.

> **Comment:** To put it quite simply, MGN-3 and AHCC are immune system boosters that compete in their own class. Our immune system is part of the last defense against cancer (see chapter on the immune system).

CHAPTER 32

How to Destroy Cancer Tumors Head-On

Comment: After you have made your body as healthy as can be, depending on the severity of your cancer, you may want to add something to directly destroy cancer tumors. I have not had any personal experience with the treatments discussed in this chapter; rather I have provided an overview of some treatments that you may want to learn more about and to which you may be exposed, depending upon the cancer that you have. However, with the exception of the following two substances, graviola and paw paw discussed immediately below, the rest of these "cancer killers", if taken long term, will damage a healthy body. Moreover, with or without cancer, improper dosing of the following items could potentially make you very sick. These substances function by actually shutting down something or stopping some action that cancer cells and tumors need to survive. As such, this causes an extra burden on the healthy cells in your body.

i) **Graviola or Soursop (*Annona Muricata*)**

Comment: Graviola is dirt cheap but hard to find. Graviola shuts down cancer cells and viruses, and is up to ten thousand times more effective than chemotherapy drugs at killing cancer cells *in vitro* (in a test tube). Graviola functions by "turning down the voltage" of cancer cells. Normal cells can operate at about 50 millivolts (mvs), but fast growing, high energy-using cancer cells need to operate at about 70 to 110 mvs, which graviola does not allow.

Comment: There was a billion dollar drug company in the United States that tried to synthesize two of the most powerful anticancer chemicals of the graviola tree for nearly seven years. Unfortunately, they could not isolate these chemicals, and consequently, had no hope of obtaining a patent, and therefore, no hope of acquiring a profit. Sadly, all testing on graviola-related compounds was abandoned. The project was shelved and the relevant findings were not published. However, one responsible researcher decided he had to blow the whistle on this natural cancer killer and released the information to certain members of the public.

Graviola, also called Brazilian pawpaw, soursop and guanabana, as well as numerous other names, refers to a particular tree or its fruit. The fruit is green and heart-shaped and is about six to eight inches (15.24 to 20.32 cm) in diameter. The tree is found in South America and on numerous tropical islands and grows best in rainforest climates.

The pulp of the fruit is popular in juices, sherbets, and smoothies. It exhibits notes of tangy and sweet. It also can be peeled and eaten, although some find the taste alone too sour. As a fruit, graviola may not prove exceptional, but it certainly has an extended history of use in ancient and now modern herbal remedies.

In early times, the leaves of the graviola were used for tea to reduce swelling of the mucus membranes (catarrh) and to treat liver disease. The black seeds were often crushed and used as a vermifuge (expels and kills internal parasites). All parts of the tree might be ground and used as a sedative or as an anticonvulsant. The fruit was used to reduce joint pain, to treat heart conditions, as a sedative, to induce labor, or to reduce coughing or flu symptoms.

http://www.wisegeek.com/what-is-graviola.htm

Graviola destroys selectively prostate, lung, breast, colon, and pancreatic cancers, leaving healthy cells intact.

In 1976, the National Cancer Institute (NCI) in United States included graviola in a plant-screening program and found that its leaves and stems were effective in attacking and destroying malignant cells. The results were part of an internal NCI report, but for some reason, were never released to the public.

Graviola has been shown to kill cancer cells *in vitro* in at least twenty laboratory tests.

In the most recent study, conducted at Catholic University of Korea earlier this year, investigators found that two compounds extracted from graviola seeds were selectively cytotoxic for breast and colon cancer cells *in vitro*, comparable with Adriamycin, a commonly used chemotherapy drug.

Another study, published in the *Journal of Natural Products*, showed that graviola not only is comparable to Adriamycin, but also graviola outperforms Adriamycin in laboratory tests. Thus, one of the graviola compounds selectively killed colon cancer cells at ten thousand times the potency of Adriamycin.

Other promising and ongoing research at Purdue University is supported by a grant from NCI. Purdue researchers recently found that leaves from the graviola tree killed cancer cells "among six human cancer cell lines" and were especially effective against prostate and pancreatic cancer cells.

In a separate study, Purdue researchers showed that extracts from the graviola leaves are extremely effective in isolating and killing lung cancer cells.

Graviola fights more than cancer. While the research on graviola has focused on its cancer-fighting effects, it also is noted that graviola has been used for centuries by medicine men in South America to treat an astonishing number of ailments. These included:

hypertension
influenza
rashes
neuralgia
arthritis
rheumatism
diarrhea
nausea
dyspepsia
ulcers
ringworm
scurvy
malaria
dysentery
palpitations
nervousness
insomnia

fever
boils
muscle spasms

http://health.centreforce.com/health/graviola.html

> **Comment:** Purdue researchers reported that the acetogenins pre-ferentially kill multidrug-resistant cancer cells by blocking the transfer of ATP, the chief source of cellular energy within the cells. ATP is needed for tumor cell energy, for growth and reproduction. ATP also is needed in more abundance in order for tumors to defend themselves from our body's natural defense mechanisms. Thus, inhibition of tumor cell energy shuts down the defense mechanisms of tumor cells. When acetogenins block access to the ATP pathway in tumor cells, they no longer have sufficient energy to sustain their life and they die.

> **Comment:** I have found graviola effective for killing cold viruses. It works very well, but it is incredibly difficult to get. It took me seven months just to find it. If you do decide to try it, remember to add a combination of probiotics in the evening (as it will also kill the good bacteria in your stomach). As well, vitamin C and CoQ10 help your cells with "energy", and are therefore, are counteractive to graviola.

ii) PawPaw Tree

> **Comment:** This is my number 1 choice for killing cancer cells because it is more potent than graviola, if you feel the need to complement your new "healthy diet".

Paw-paw is clearly more powerful than graviola for the treatment of cancer, if the quality of the processing is comparable, since the acetognins in graviola have only single rings whereas the acetogenins in paw-paw have several double rings (e.g., bullatacin), which make them more powerful.

Paw-paw works (and I assume graviola as well) by slowing down or stopping the production of ATP. This, in turn, lowers the voltage of the cell. For normal cells, there is plenty of ATP, thus, lowering the level of ATP has no effect on these cells. However, with cancer cells, due to the way they create energy (by fermentation), ATP is far more critical. When the ATP level, and therefore, the energy of the cell decrease to a critical level, the cancer cells falls apart. The residual pieces of the dead cancer cell are "lysed", and I assume, are similar to other apoptosis (programmed cell death) killed cells. If that is the case, then these residual pieces are literally "*eaten*" by other cells.

However, because the cancer cells in a cancer patient are frequently clustered together, a large amount of lysis can occur within a cancer patient such that high levels of clustered debris cannot be eaten by surrounding cells. Such a situation is especially dangerous for lung cancer patients and brain cancer patients where a clustered amount of residual cancer cell debris can be very dangerous.

http://cancertutor.com/Cancer/Graviola.html

iii) Sodium Bicarbonate a.k.a. Baking Soda

> **Comment:** Dr. T. Simoncini believes that cancer is caused predominantly by *Candida* (and the bad toxins given off by their actions). He suggests that sodium bicarbonate (baking soda) is the cure for cancer. As well as killing the bad Candida bacteria, baking soda is extremely alkaline. If you recall, Candida can disrupt your whole body and cancer cannot survive in high alkaline environment. However, killing Candida and making the body alkaline are only two parts of the equation and will only work to their full potential if the other pieces of the "arch" are functioning properly as well.

http://www.curenaturalicancro.com/2-cause-cancer.html

Is it difficult in a laboratory to show that tumors decrease through bicarbonate?

No, there are a hundred tests that can demonstrate this effect, but in a wrong manner. One attributes to bicarbonate an antitumor effect because of its alkalinizing qualities, but the bicarbonate is effective because it eliminates the fungus. The other products (alkalinizing matters) do not work (or very little) against the fungus.

Dr Mark Sircus Ac OMD and Dr Simoncini

http://www.curenaturalicancro.com/cancer-therapy-faq.html

> **Comment:** Another "remedy" for cancer revolves around reversing Candida and alkalizing the body. It works very well in a test tube; therefore, the only variances in the human body could be cellular toxicity and ability of baking soda to access and attack the fungus directly. Given

these factors, I suggest that the use of baking soda is restricted to the fighting of certain cancers only, rather than long term prevention (since it only addresses two of several cancer issues, pH and Candida).

iv) Canabis and Cannabinoids

Comment: There is a gentleman in Nova Scotia who attempted to reverse cancer using hemp oil. He went to jail for the "possession, growing and selling" of marijuana, even though he gave it to several people he knows in the form of "oil" and for free. Many of these people had their cancer go into remission and speak about the cannabis as their savior.

http://www.cannabisculture.com/articles/5081.html

Cannabinoids May Inhibit Cancer Cell Invasion

Science Daily (Dec. 27, 2007) Cannabinoids may suppress tumor invasion in highly invasive cancers, according to a study published online December 25 in the *Journal of the National Cancer Institute*.

Cannabinoids, the active components in marijuana, are used to reduce the side effects of cancer treatment, such as pain, weight loss, and vomiting. However, there is increasing evidence that cannabinoids may also inhibit tumor cell growth, although the underlying mechanism(s) for their inhibitory effects are unknown.

Robert Ramer, PhD, and Burkhard Hinz, PhD, of the University of Rostock in Germany investigated whether and by what mechanism Cannabinoids inhibit tumor cell invasion.

He found that cannabinoids suppressed tumor cell invasion and stimulated the expression of TIMP-1, an inhibitor of a group of enzymes that are involved in tumor cell invasion.

"To our knowledge, this is the first report of TIMP-1-dependent anti-invasive effects of Cannabinoids. This signaling pathway may play an important role in the antimetastatic action of Cannabinoids, whose potential therapeutic benefit in the treatment of highly invasive cancers should be addressed in clinical trials," the authors write.

Journal of the National Cancer Institute, via EurekAlert!, a service of AAAS

Marijuana Compound Shows Promise in Fighting Breast Cancer

Science Daily (Nov. 26, 2007) A compound found in *Cannabis* may prove to be effective at helping stop the spread of breast cancer cells throughout the body.

The study, by scientists at the California Pacific Medical Center Research Institute, is raising hope that CBD, a compound found in *Cannabis sativa*, could be the first non-toxic agent to show promise in treating metastatic forms of breast cancer.

"Right now we have a limited range of options in treating aggressive forms of cancer," says Sean D. McAllister, PhD, a cancer researcher at CPMCRI and the lead author of the study. "Those treatments, such as chemotherapy, can be effective but they can also be extremely toxic and difficult for patients. This compound offers the hope of a non-toxic therapy that could achieve the same results without any of the painful side effects."

The researchers used CBD to inhibit the activity of a gene called Id-1, which is believed to be responsible for the aggressive spread of cancer cells throughout the body, away from the original tumor site.

"We know that Id-1 is a key regulator of the spread of breast cancer," says Pierre-Yves Desprez, PhD, a cancer researcher at CPMCRI and the senior author of the study. "We also know that Id-1 has also been found at higher levels in other forms of cancer. So what is exciting about this study is that if CBD can inhibit Id-1 in breast cancer cells, then it may also prove effective at stopping the spread of cancer cells in other forms of the disease, such as colon and brain or prostate cancer."

However, the researchers point out that while their findings are promising they are not a recommendation for people with breast cancer to smoke marijuana. They say it is highly unlikely that effective concentrations of CBD could be reached by smoking *Cannabis*. And while CBD is not psychoactive it is still considered a Schedule 1 drug.

This study was recently published in the journal, *Molecular Cancer Therapeutics*.

The study was primarily funded by the California Breast Cancer Research Program.

California Pacific Medical Center

http://www.newswise.com./

http://www.sciencedaily.com/releases/2007/11/071123211703.htm

> **Comment:** If one were so inclined to make hemp oil, it should only take about ten minutes to find out how on the Internet or YouTube.

v) Methylglyoxal a.k.a Retine

> **Comment:** Normally produced in the body, methylglyoxal affects cancer cells by shutting down the ability of the cancer cells to produce ATP (similar to graviola and pawpaw). By shutting down a cancer cell's ability to produce ATP, growth and cell division are halted.

Explaining the mechanism of action, some scientists reported that "Cancer cells required a large amount of energy-providing substance called ATP (adenosine-5-triphosphate) for survival."

"Methylglyoxal inactivates the enzyme (glyceraldehydes-3-Phosphate Dehydrogenase) needed for ATP production in cancer cells, thereby starving them to death. Normal cells remain unaffected."

Manju Ray said that chemists knew about the methylglyoxal molecule for about four decades and that its anti-cancer effects in animals also had been studied. "But surprisingly, no one bothered to initiate further research leading to human trials."

The researchers said concern in some quarters about safety of methylglyoxal were not borne out from the clinical trials, which showed that in combination with a protective agent like ascorbic acid and vitamins, the drug methylglyoxal had no major toxic effect.

They said there was scope for further enhancing the drug's efficacy.

Hindustan Times, Hyderabad, May 28, 2001

Dr. Szent-Gyorgyi explained that he and Dr. Egyud found that retine (methylglyoxal) stops the growth of cancer cells without poisoning other cells. When retine is present in sufficient concentration, cell division cannot occur while vital cellular processes go on unhindered. The article goes on, "And what is a good bit of luck, and not my cleverness," the white-haired scientist pointed out, "is that if a cancer cell cannot grow, it dies by itself." According to the researchers, retine can be produced normally by the body and, when it is, it prevents the growth of existing cancer cells. But the body can lose its ability to produce this substance. "Putting the retine back in the body, just as we put insulin back into a diabetic's body, can stop the growth of cancer." The scientists at Woods Hole found that "cancer cells are much more sensitive to retine than normal ones, and so cancer cells may be inhibited specifically."

http://www.arrowheadhealthworks.com/Retine_C.html

In Koch's book, *Survival Factor in Neoplastic and Viral Diseases*, there is a series of photos of an infant girl diagnosed with inoperable liver cancer who had a protrusion of the abdomen, which got less and less until she is shown as a healthy young girl. And many other users have experienced similar results.

The formulations trigger a chain reaction in every cell on a molecular level and tap into the body's infinite capacity to reverse any disease. Dr. Koch called his primary remedy the Synthetic Survival Reagent, and used it successfully for treating cancers, allergies, polio and infectious diseases. He postulated that it worked against pathogens because the increased oxidation initiated by it would kill the disease causing pathogens in the cells.

They also help to deal with the damaging effects of free radicals throughout the body. In a sense, causing a chain reaction at the DNA level among all existing free radicals will nullify them so that they cannot cause disease. When you take them along with other free radical scavengers, the damaging effects from the vast amounts of free radicals we are exposed to in this polluted world can be greatly negated. It can bring about dramatic changes in the cells because it normalizes DNA function with the removal of free radicals and subsequently affects how cells replicate.

In addition, it is theorized to be able to interfere with the DNA of pathogenic micro organisms and cancer cells to shut down their replication, and thus cause them to die. An MD who worked with Koch's formulations said that he found it to be about 80% effective against cancer.

As a historical note, in Germany they have been used to treat many different diseases. German authorities on these remedies say that they treat cancer, HIV, chronic infectious diseases, auto-immune diseases, and can be used as a replacement for vaccinations of diseases such as chicken pox and measles, and basically treat any and all disease. (Heart disease is intimately connected to free radical damage and bacterial infections.) Because the TMT molecules are extremely small, it has no problem working on diseases of the brain.

Methylglyoxal, if you remember, literally tells cancer cells to stop their abnormally high replication rate. Cancer cells are revved up way past the red line, so to speak, so when it comes to cell replication, they replicate many times faster than normal cells. Methylglyoxal is missing from those cells. TMT uses a very slight amount of methylglyoxal that starts a self-replicating process, causing the cell to repair itself as methylglyoxal is introduced to the cell and passes on to restore the methylglyoxal in another cell, causing a cascade of cellular repair and a stopping of uncontrolled replication. As Dr. Szent-Gyorgyi discovered, when cancer cells cannot replicate in an uncontrolled fashion, they die. And of course, at the same time, as these remedies turn off the replication of cancer cells, they initiate the repair of respiratory enzymes from cell to cell.

TMT is Dr. Koch's full range of five different homeopathic formulations of glyoxal and methylglyoxal work together to stimulate your body to create more methylglyoxal in the cells. They have been used for fifty years in Germany and have proven again and again to be quite powerful in their cancer-fighting effects.

http://www.cancerfightingstrategies.com/methylglyoxal.html

vi) Cesium Science and Cesium Therapy

> **Comment:** An acidic body holds less oxygen. A body deprived of oxygen will grow cancer very quickly. Conversely, cancer cannot survive in a high oxygen environment. Cesium is a soft, silvery-gold alkali metal, which is known to make the body more alkaline and therefore hold more oxygen. Two pieces of the cancer equation that we know will reduce cancer's ability to survive. Cesium is also known to reduce the ability of cancer cells to ferment sugar for energy (thus, starving them to death).

Almost seventy-five years ago, Otto Warburg was awarded two Nobel Prizes for his theories that cancer is caused by impaired cell respiration due to a lack of oxygen at the cellular level. According to Warburg, damaged cell respiration causes fermentation, resulting in hyperacidity at the cellular level. Briefly, a normal cell undergoes an adverse change when it can no longer take up oxygen to convert glucose into energy by oxidation. In the absence of oxygen, the cell reverts to a primitive nutritional program to sustain itself, converting glucose (blood sugar) by fermentation. The lactic acid produced by fermentation lowers the cell pH (acid/alkaline balance) and destroys the ability of DNA and RNA to control cell division, and cancer cells begin to multiply unchecked. The lactic acid simultaneously causes intense local pain and destroys cell enzymes. Therefore, cancer appears as a rapidly growing outer cell mass with a core of dead cells.

In 1984, Keith Brewer, PhD (Physics) translated Warburg's theories into a practical, cost-efficient treatment protocol for cancer. Brewer successfully treated thirty patients with various cancers, using cesium, nature's most alkaline mineral. The results of Brewer's work—all thirty patients survived!

Dr. Brewer noted that the element also apparently retards aging. After taking cesium daily for five years, he reported he was still more vigorous than when he began. He was ninety-two by that time. This is consistent with research being done with treatment of chronic fatigue. An increase of the alkalinity in the body by 0.6 pH increases the amount of oxygen in the blood by almost 70%. It is only logical that this would increase one's energy and mental alertness and help avert degenerative diseases. It also is a healthier energy source than caffeine, candy, drugs or alcohol.

In 1996, Neal Deoul provided financing that enabled T-UP Inc. to become a primary distributor of cesium and concentrated aloe vera. Hundreds of cancer patients experienced remarkable results using cesium and T-UP aloe vera in their battles against cancer.

Cesium, a naturally occurring alkaline element, has been shown to affect the cancer cell in two ways. First, cesium limits the cellular uptake of the nutrient glucose, starving the cancer cell and diminishing fermentation. Second, cesium raises the cell pH to the range of 8.0 neutralizing the weak lactic acid and stopping pain within twelve to twenty-four hours. A pH range of 8.0 is a deadly environment for the cancer cell; the cancer cell dies within a few days and is absorbed and eliminated by the body.

The science of high pH therapy (drastically changing the acid/alkaline balance of the cell):

By the late 1970s, mass spectrographic and isotope studies had shown that tumor cells exhibit a preference for the uptake of certain alkaline minerals. These included potassium, rubidium, and especially cesium. Furthermore, specific antioxidants (i.e., vitamin C and zinc) were shown to enhance the uptake of these alkaline minerals by the cancer cell.

A normal cell is surrounded by a membrane, which selectively allows materials to flow in and out. Oxygen and nutrients, such as glucose, flow in. Waste products of cellular chemistry flow out. The cells are protected by the immune system; a well-functioning immune system is the best defense against the formation of cancer cells. When environmental toxins (carcinogens) overwhelm the immune system, the entire program is compromised. The cell membrane is affected first, losing its ability to exchange oxygen (respiration); the cell then reverts to a primitive survival mechanism, fermentation. The newly formed (anaerobic) cancer cell cannot be repaired (fermentation is not reversible). The cell is now out of control and must be destroyed as rapidly as possible.

It is interesting to note that in areas of the world where there is a high cesium content in the soil, cancer is virtually unknown, such as for the Hopi Indians of Arizona, the Hunza of North Pakistan, and the Indians of Central and South America. These observations suggest the possibility of a vitamin/mineral/antioxidant formulation containing cesium in an amount equal to that found in the soil of cancer-free habitats could be a powerful new tool to help slow down and even reverse the present cancer epidemic.

http://www.angelfire.com/az/sthurston/stop_cancer_cells_with_cesium.html

> **Comment:** Cesium is the most alkaline and electropositive element. Electropositivity is a measure of an element's ability to donate electrons. The donating of electrons, as you will remember from earlier, is an ability portrayed by antioxidants (which go hand in hand with alkalinity). Although cesium alludes to positive responses, it is still a heavy metal and the only way I would use it personally is if I had brain cancer as most metals are able to cross the blood brain barrier due to size. However, I do not suggest cesium for long term good health, as I suspect chronic ingestion of metals could have cumulative effects.

vii) Enzyme L-Asparaginase

> **Comment:** This drug is merely for breaking down tumors immediately. It would not be positive factors in long term good health. Asparaginase breaks down the amino acid (L-asparagine)

required for DNA synthesis and cell survival. It is capable of "shutting down" cancer tumors. Conversely, most healthy cells are capable of synthesizing asparagine from glutamine. Therefore, healthy cells will not be as drastically affected as the cancer cells (that cannot perform this synthesis). This works well for leukemia (cancer of the blood). But not very well for brain cancer, as it is not possible for asparaginase to cross the blood brain barrier.

Anonymous. Asparaginase: Drug Information. In: Rose BD, editor. UpToDate Wellesley, Massachusetts: UpToDate 14.2; 2006

McEvoy GK. *AHFS* Drug Information. 2006, Bethesda, Maryland: American Society of Health-System Pharmacists, Inc.; 2006. p. 932-4.

Graham ML. Pegaspargase: a review of clinical studies. Adv Drug Delivery *Rev* 2003; 55(10):1293-302.

Mechanism of Action

The rationale behind asparaginase is that it takes advantage of the fact that ALL leukemic cells are unable to synthesize the nonessential amino acid asparagine, whereas normal cells are able to make their own asparagine; thus, leukemic cells require high amount of asparagine. These leukemic cells depend on circulating asparagine. Asparaginase, however, catalyzes the conversion of L-asparagine to aspartic acid and ammonia. This deprives the leukemic cell of circulating asparagine.

http://en.wikipedia.org/wiki/Asparaginase

Protein Anticancer Agent: Enzyme L-Asparaginase:

In the 1950s, a biochemical difference in metabolism related to the amino acid asparagine was found. Normal cells apparently can synthesize asparagine while leukemia cells cannot. If leukemia cells are deprived of asparagine, they will eventually die. In an almost unrecognized and parallel discovery, it was found that blood serum from guinea pigs and other South American rodents had antileukemia properties. The enzyme L-asparaginase was eventually identified as the anticancer agent. L-asparaginase was isolated and tested successfully on human leukemias. Eventually, the enzyme asparaginase was also found and isolated from the bacteria *E. coli.*

If the enzyme L-asparaginase is given to humans, various types of leukemias can be controlled. Tumor cells, more specifically lymphatic tumor cells, require huge amounts of asparagines to keep up with their rapid, malignant growth. This means they use both asparagine from the diet as well as what they can make themselves (which is limited) to satisfy their large asparagines demand.

http://www.elmhurst.edu/~chm/vchembook/655cancer.html

> **Comment:** It has been reported that tiredness and lack of energy sometimes occur with this drug. Probably because it stops a "positive" reaction in your body, which is not at all my first choice for reversing cancer because it falls into the category of killing tumors immediately and not reversing the cause of the tumor. Although I suspect it would be useful for short term use and an immediate response from tumors.

viii) Sodium Dichloroacetate a.k.a. DCA and Chlorine Dioxide a.k.a. MMS

> **Comment:** DCA and MMS are thought to attack cancer (and viruses) directly affecting nothing else. Although, that being said, I feel I should point out these are not *"original"* components of the human body, and therefore, are not required to facilitate a healthy body. In addition to this, a portion of both DCA and MMS is chlorine, which, as has been discussed earlier, is good for killing bacteria, moulds and viruses, but not so good for the human body. It should be noted however, that the portion that is not chlorine is oxygen. Hopefully, you remember from an earlier chapter on oxygen that it has detoxifying abilities due to its weak outer shell.

> This method of attacking cancer has its limitations for two reasons. First, it will not address the underlying "causes" of the cancer nor "rebalance" the body chemistry. Second, for DCA and MMS to be effective, their doses must be continuously increased until you cannot tolerate them anymore; namely they may eventually cause nausea, diarrhea and/or vomiting as part of the cleansing process. However, this therapeutic approach does appear to have some potential, especially when one adds DMSO, which appears to increase the absorption potential of DCA into the cells.

Sodium Dichloroacetate (DCA)

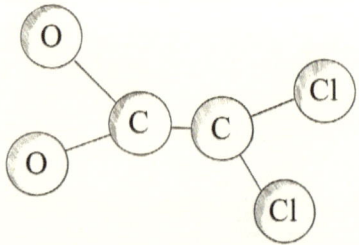

Sodium Dichloroacetate molecule

MMS/Chlorine Dioxide ($CLO_{2\ ion}$)

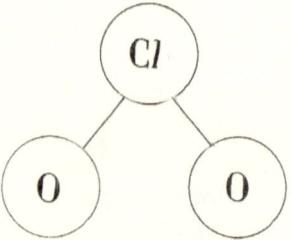

http://www.getmms.org/images/ClO2-image.jpg

From the University of Alberta: Small Molecule Offers Big Hope Against Cancer

DCA is an odorless, colorless, inexpensive, relatively non-toxic, small molecule. And researchers at the University of Alberta believe it may soon be used as an effective treatment for many forms of cancer. Dr. Evangelos Michelakis, a professor at the U of A, Department of Medicine, found that dichloroacetate (DCA) causes regression of several cancers, including lung, breast, and brain tumors. Michelakis *et al* have published their results in the journal *Cancer Cell*.

Scientists and doctors have used DCA for decades to treat children with inborn errors of metabolism due to mitochondrial diseases. Mitochondria, the energy producing units in cells, have been connected with cancer since the 1930s, when researchers first noticed that these organelles dysfunction when cancer is present.

Until recently, researchers believed that cancer-affected mitochondria are permanently damaged and that this damage is the result, not the cause, of the cancer. But Michelakis questioned this belief and began testing DCA, which activates a critical mitochondrial enzyme, as a way to "revive" the mitochondria of cancer cells. The results astounded him. Michelakis and his colleagues found that DCA normalized the mitochondrial function in many cancers, showing that their function was actively suppressed by the cancer but was not permanently damaged by it. More importantly, they found that the normalization of mitochondrial function resulted in a significant decrease in tumor growth both in test tubes and in animal models. Also, they noted that DCA, unlike most currently used chemotherapies, did not have any effects on normal, non-cancerous tissues.

"I think DCA can be selective for cancer because it attacks a fundamental process in cancer development that is unique to cancer cells," Michelakis said. "Cancer cells actively suppress their mitochondria, which alters their metabolism, and this appears to offer cancer cells a significant advantage in growth compared to normal cells, as well as protection from many standard chemotherapies. Because mitochondria regulate cell death or "apoptosis", cancer cells can thus achieve resistance to apoptosis, and this appears to be reversed by DCA."

"One of the really exciting things about this compound is that it might be able to treat many different forms of cancer, because all forms of cancer suppress mitochondrial function; in fact, this is why most cancers can be detected by tests like positron emission tomography (PET), which detects the unique metabolic profile of cancer compared to normal cells," added Michelakis, the Canada Research Chair in Pulmonary Hypertension.

Another encouraging thing about DCA is that, being so small, it is easily absorbed in the body, and after oral intake, it can reach areas in the body that other drugs cannot, making it possible to treat brain cancers, for example.

Also, because DCA has been used in both healthy people and sick patients with mitochondrial diseases, researchers already know that it is a relatively non-toxic molecule that can be immediately tested in patients with cancer.

Furthermore, the DCA compound is not patented and not owned by any pharmaceutical company, and, therefore, would likely be an inexpensive drug to administer, Michelakis added.

However, as DCA is not patented, Michelakis is concerned that it may be difficult to find funding from private investors to test DCA in clinical trials. He is grateful for the support he has already received from publicly funded agencies, such as the Canadian Institutes for Health Research (CIHR), and he is hopeful such support will continue and allow him to conduct clinical trials of DCA on cancer patients.

"This preliminary research is encouraging and offers hope to thousands of Canadians and all those around the world who are afflicted by cancer, as it accelerates our understanding of and action around targeted cancer treatments," said Dr. Philip Branton, Scientific Director of the CIHR Institute of Cancer.

http://www.encognitive.com/node/2853

DCA has now been approved for a trial in brain cancer patients in Canada. The researchers have raised $800,000 in public donations to fund the trial.

http://scienceblog.cancerresearchuk.org/2010/05/12/potential-cancer-drug-dca-tested-in-early-trials/

> **Comment:** This seems to be to be pretty harsh on the body, but it is very easy to find, and you can make it at home. It has also been reported to attack viral diseases like AIDS as well.

Medicine or food taken orally goes into the stomach where stomach acids will extract chlorine dioxide, which is then picked up by the red blood cell (known as the "bus driver", who, fortunately, is colorblind and underpaid). His normal job description is to carry oxygen to the different cells in the body. However, since chlorine dioxide looks the same and has the same signature as oxygen, the "bus driver" is fooled into transporting chlorine dioxide to the different awaiting cells. The working nature of the chlorine dioxide ion is very volatile when it comes into contact with pathogens. It is agreed that no pathogen can develop a resistance to it. When a chlorine dioxide ion contacts a harmful pathogen, it instantly accepts five electrons. Perhaps it is more descriptive is to say that the chlorine dioxide ion instantly tears off five electrons. This is an extremely fast chemical reaction, which is, in essence, an explosion on a microscopic level! The pathogen basically is oxidized by chlorine dioxide ions, and as part of an action, the chlorine becomes harmless chloride (table salt) that is easily eliminated from the body.

In summary, the immune system uses chlorine dioxide, a chemical needed to destroy illnesses, by sending first the "bus driver" to pick it up in the food factory, and transport it and finally deposit it to the immune system, which, on receiving the deposit of chlorine dioxide, goes through the process of myeloberoxidase, making it into a deadly instrument or carrier. On impact with a pathogen, it, in a milli-second, produces hypochlorous acid, which destroys the enemy cells. Hypochlorous acid is the weapon that the white blood cell uses to kill parasites, bacteria, fungi, viruses, tumor cells, natural killer cells and waste products. Hypochlorous acid has the ability to add eighty electrons instead of the usual five electrons to the white blood cell, turning the usual hand grenade into an atomic bomb, ensuring that the white blood cell has enough energy to return to the red blood cell to pick up another atomic bomb. All this happens within a three minute time space to eradicate diseases.

In most cases of illness, the immune system has been depleted because of our lifestyle and eating habits, as well as chemical intervention into our natural products (preservatives) and GM foods. The body does not receive the correct nutrients to enable the manufacturing of ClO2 ions, resulting in the white blood cells not having the ability to produce hypochlorous acid.

http://www.cancercure.co.za/

ix) Zeolite

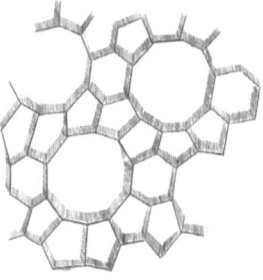

Zeolite

Comment: Zeolite is another agent used to break down cancer tumors. In order for zeolite to work effectively on cancer, zeolite also must be taken in a dose that causes one to feel ill (similar to DCA or MMS). Such a heavy cleansing is bound to cause a disruption in the body's normal functions, however, I do not recommend this in practice. Zeolite cleansing does not maintain consistency with the premise of *"balance"*. To me, zeolite is more of a super cleanse that will wash cancer right out of the body, in what I suspect, will not be a very gentle way.

Zeolites come from natural "volcanic rocks" with a very complex and unique structure made up of crystalline (shaped like honeycomb) object that gets to the cells of your body and helps trap and remove the heavy toxins and metals in a safe, natural way. And because it is only one of the few minerals in nature that is negatively charged, zeolite actually attracts and draws the harmful metals and toxins in your body to it, and then captures and cages them safely so your body can help remove them!

Cellular zeolite concentrates on two main health benefits. Detoxification is essential for anyone who is trying to regain his/her health back and to prevent or overcome most diseases. But the problem is, this is only half of the solution. You have to be able to rebuild your weakened body system by putting in the vital minerals, foods, nutrients, and supplements. Natural cellular defense with liquid zeolite will help detoxify your body of some of the heavy metals and toxins such as lead and mercury.

Liquid Zeolite Benefits the Body Beyond Detoxification

It removes carcinogens, toxins, and heavy metals from your body.

It helps nutrients to flow throughout the body easier.

It allows your body to remove free radicals before doing potential damage.

It balances your body's pH. It lowers blood sugar by absorbing glucose. It helps fight common viruses and traps and removes them naturally from the body.

It has the ability to reduce acid reflux. It helps fight asthma, migraines, and allergies.

http://www.liquidcellularzeolites.com/

Zeolite Fights Cancer in Several Ways:

It chelates and removes heavy metals, pesticides, herbicides, and other toxins from your body. It does this in a hierarchical manner. It is most attracted to lead, mercury, cadmium, arsenic and other heavy metals, but also chelates pesticides, herbicides, plastics, and so forth. It acts as a natural trap of viral particles, thereby stopping the production of the viruses.

Because it traps toxins in its molecular structure, it detoxifies without overloading the detoxification system in your body. As toxins are an underlying cause of almost all cancers, taking zeolite on a regular basis is an excellent cancer preventative, especially as it can kill any cancer cells that may develop.

In addition, zeolite traps free radicals in its molecular structure so it acts as a free radical scavenger too. It will also help to normalize body pH, and helps boost the immune system by increasing the levels of CD4 immune system molecules.

One Additional Benefit:

Ammonia is a toxin that has no place in a healthy body. Thousands of people with liver and kidney disease die every year from too much ammonia in their blood. The average person can handle low levels of ammonia in his/her blood, but even a low level adds stress to the immune system and compromises health.

Most ammonia forms in the body when protein is broken down by unfriendly bacteria in the intestines. It is also produced by parasites, yeasts and moulds. These organisms produce ammonia both as a waste product and as a mechanism to keep their host (your body) in an unhealthy state. And as Candida yeast is almost always overgrown and infecting the whole body of someone with cancer, you may well have high levels of ammonia in your body.

A healthy liver converts ammonia into urea, which is then eliminated in urine. A benefit of dietary zeolite is its ability to remove ammonia directly from your body, which means less stress on your liver and kidneys. That is a big bonus for your health if your liver is weak. Of course, reduced ammonia also is a bonus for healthy digestion. Pathogens and parasites are weakened, and beneficial bacteria can better recolonize.

For this reason, the use of dietary zeolite may be very helpful if your liver is not working properly. Ammonia that remains unprocessed because the liver is not working up to par can enter the bloodstream and invade the central nervous system, causing many dangerous effects. Even your brain can be affected. In advanced cases of liver disease, for example, the ammonia may cause at first a mild mental aberration, which can progress to coma and, ultimately, death. Increased levels of ammonia in the blood are characteristic of liver failure.

http://www.cancer-prevention.net/

CHAPTER 33

Conclusions and Implications

Hopefully, I have provided you with some new perspectives and understanding on how you might prevent and/or reverse cancer. However, I cannot stress this enough, you still need to do your own research. But I encourage you to become informed and think for yourself, albeit with the guidance of your doctor or naturopath, or preferably both. This book represents only miniature tidbits of information on each topic. What I have learned is that preventing cancer long term is a lifestyle. We need to keep things in balance. We can overdue anything. If you have cancer, then something has tipped the scale in the wrong direction. How you get back in balance lies in your ability to tip the scale back in the right direction of good health. Just like building a house, we know that there are many pieces required and more than one way to do it. I have now found thirteen cancer clinics (see appendix 1) that will help you do exactly that. The information is out there. Do not feel trapped into using your doctor, surgery or pharmaceuticals as your only source of remediation.

After all my readings, I have concluded that my cancer equation first started with acidosis, Candida, stress and toxic overload. I also smoked and was not getting enough oxygen into my body. I worked shifts and was not sleeping enough. I ate an acidic (poor) diet. I did not put enough vitamins, minerals, nutrients and essential fats into my body for proper repairing, immune system strength or proper blood pH. The reason I did not get better after removing my kidney was because my body was already very weak. I did not address any of these cancer causing problems until it was too late. But it is not too late.

I am reminded of the old adage, "Rome was not built in a day". Everything in my life that has been worthwhile has taken me a long time. If you try to do all the things at once, you will, in all probability, fail. Start with one thing each week. Then add another the week after. Then add another the week after that. Pretty soon, you will feel like the superhuman you deserve to feel like. The key lesson is to be healthy so that you can prevent and reverse cancer, in its simplified form it is to remove the cause(s) of cancer. What you put into your body will be the building blocks to the masterpiece that is your body. Balance is the key. Prevention and the reversal of cancer are one and the same. Cancer cannot survive in a healthy body. AND there are several less damaging (and less expensive) ways to destroy cancer cells other than chemo and radiation therapy.

1st   Remember that free radicals (that promote cancer) and antioxidants must be balanced equally. You cannot avoid continuous free radical formations. So in order to maintain balance, you need to add antioxidants to your diet.

2nd   In order for your body to destroy cancer cells, your immune system must be strong and functioning properly. I currently use colostrum, but for cancer, you may want to try MGN-3 or AHCC as an adjunct to your immune system.

3rd   Your lymphatic system, which runs in parallel to your bloodstream to wash some of the junk and garbage out of your body, must also be functioning. (Remember that your lymphatic system has no heart (pump) like your bloodstream, so muscle contraction on a daily basis is mandatory!).

4th   Next, you need to maintain your blood pH around 7.45. An acidic pH can cause cancer, and conversely, cancer cannot survive in a high alkaline environment. This will be determined by your food and liquid intake and stress.

5th   After that, it seems redundant to say that detoxifying is crucial. Toxic overload can cause cancer. There are many things that your body will store and not remove by itself. Consider a heavy metal cleanse and a colon cleanse.

6th   After that, your body requires a healthy amount of oxygen. Learn proper breathing techniques. (Cancer cannot survive in a high oxygen environment.) Your body requires the right "fuel".

7th   The right "fuel" also includes vitamins, minerals, macrominerals, amino acids, and lots of clean water (preferably alkaline). Learn about Gerson therapy.

8th   In order for most of this to happen, your digestive system must be fully functioning (with probiotics). If your digestive system is not functioning properly, you will not absorb enough of those nutrients, and Candida (which can cause cancer) can eventually take over.

9th The sun gives you energy. Do not be afraid of it, just don't overdo it. Sunshine is also the only way to convert cholesterol into real vitamin D.

10th Once these pieces are in place, I suggest working on the psychological aspect of life and getting rid of stress.

11th After that, try going to an acupuncture doctor. Acupuncture doctors see the body as a "whole" and, as such will work to assist your body in healing itself.

12th Consider getting your hormones checked. They must be proportionately balanced for proper physiological and psychological function.

13th Be aware of the electromagnetic forces in your close proximity. As you slowly add (or remove) each one of these things to your regimen, you will begin to feel better and better. If you do some of these things really well or most of them halfway, cancer will never be able to survive in your body.

14th If you are diagnosed with cancer, you may wish to learn more about destroying the tumor(s) directly. Consider further reading on graviola or pawpaw, cesium, sodium bicarbonate, MMS, DCA, cannabinoids, L-asparaginase, methylglyoxal (retine), colloidal silver, GEMM therapy or zoelite to see which one may best suit you.

15th Or you might consider contacting one of the many cancer clinics that no one told me about. They will tell you more about how to detoxify, become alkaline and strengthen your body with proper nutrition.

If you decide to learn more about these things, you will undoubtedly bump into more ways of reversing cancer as there are many. Just remember the premise of all the approaches: Return the body to its natural state of good health and balance. Cancer cannot survive in a healthy body.

The cells in your body do not have miniwatches. Time is not the main destroyer of our bodies, it is the garbage we put into them and the internal stresses we cause ourselves. We were born in a state of exquisite perfection, the trick of longevity is to keep it there.

As for me, I am now doing fantastic. Most days I feel better than I did when I was twenty. Along with regular exercise, I stick mostly to my "juice" diet of lots of berries, goji, noni, acai, mangosteen, cacao, gotu kola, spirulina and proteins in the blender every morning. I usually add a banana, apple, or pear for taste as well. Melatonin, DHEA, 5HTP, GABA, maca root and tribulus to help me maintain my hormone balance. (Please do not do this without supervision or becoming very, very well informed. Remember, I am missing a major hormone producer, my adrenal gland. Most days I also take CoQ10, L-arginine, L-tyrosine, colostrum (an immune system booster) and probiotics. I undergo acupuncture every two weeks and I listen to binaural beats for relaxation almost every day. In the winter I go tanning sometimes; and in the summer I get as much sun as I can. I never use sunscreen (not even on holidays). I have done several months of colon and heavy metal cleanses. I have purchased an air purifier, a 93% oxygen machine, a water ionizer that makes water with a pH of 10.5 and a foot detox machine. Eventually, I will buy myself a magnetic mattress. There is also a filter on my shower and even my plants do not get tap water.

A few other secrets but come on, I have got to keep something to myself. I have my cognitive function back along with lots of energy and very little pain. My back, even three years later, is still causing problems. I deal with subluxation of the spine (my disks shift out of place) on a daily basis. Fortunately, I almost have that one beat too.

Sometimes I do still sleep a lot, and my one kidney cannot take a lot of stress. I'll always regret finding all this information out at the eleventh hour, but in the end, I would do it all again. It was worth being there in order to get to where I am now. Cancer has increased my perception, understanding, and awareness. Colors are brighter, food has more flavor and I enjoy life more. It is now, so much more obvious that every moment of existence is a gift to be cherished to its fullest.

Appendix 1

Cancer Clinics:

Medicine of H.O.P.E.,
1215 E Brown Rd #2, Mesa AZ 85203
Phone: 480-668-1448
Toll Free: 1-877-668-1448
http://medicineofhope.com/home

Advanced Medical Group,
5744 Tablerock Dr., El Paso, TX 79912
Phone: 915-581-2273
E-mail: questions@amg-health.com
www.amg-health.com

Hospital Santa Monica (Donsbach Clinic)
Rosarita Beach, Mexico
Phone: 800-359-6547 or 619-427-3007
http://www.donsbach.com

Oasis of Hope Hospital USA
Phone: 1-888-500-HOPE or 619-690-8400
Fax: 619-690-8410
E-mail: care@oasisofhope.com

Saint Joseph Medical Center
Phone: 1-877-943-4673
http://www.doctorofhope.com.mx/

Hope4Cancer
Phone: Tel. 1-888-544-5993
http://www.hope4cancer.com/contact/contact-hope4cancer.html

Camelot Cancer Care
Phone: 918-493-1011
http://www.camelotcancercare.com/index.html

Gerson Institute/Cancer Curing Society
1572 Second Avenue, San Diego, CA 92101
Phone: 619-685-5353/888-443-7766 (US only)
Toll: 800-838-2256 (US and Canada)
Fax: 619-685-5363
http://www.gerson.org/

Reno Integrative Medical Center
6110 Plumas St. Ste. B Reno, Nevada 89519
Phone: 775-829-1009 or 800-994-1009
http://www.renointegrativemedicalcenter.com/

The Budwig Center
Phone: +34-952-381-447 Cell/Mobile +34-677-026-818
E-mail: budwigcenter@gmail.com
http://www.budwigcenter.com/contacts.php

Alpha Medical Clinic
Phone: 1-800-359-6547
http://alphamedicalclinic.com/Home.aspx

Hawaii Gerson Therapy Retreat
Hawaii Naturopathic Retreat Center Inc.
17-502 Ipuaiwaha
Keaau Hawaii 96749
Telephone: 808-982-8202
E-mail: gerson@mindyourbody.info
www.gersonhawaii.us
& www.mindyourbody.info
http://www.gersonhawaii.us/contact.html

NatureWorksBest.com
Naturopathic Medical Doctors of Arizona
1250 East Baseline Road, Suite 205
Tempe, AZ 85283
Phone: 480-839-2800
http://www.natureworksbest.com/

This website has an even longer list of clinics to choose from

http://www.cancertutor.com/Other/Clinics.html

APPENDIX 2

MOSS'S FIRST pH CHART

Ideal Blood pH 7.2-7.4 (at birth 7.44)

ALKALIZING VEGETABLES
Alfalfa pH 8 Asparagus pH8.5
Barley Grass
Beets pH 7.5
Beet Greens Bell Pepper 7.5
Broccoli pH7.5 Brussel Sprouts
Cabbage
Carrot pH 8
Cauliflower
Celery pH 8
Chard Greens Chives
Chlorella
Collard Greens
Cucumber
Dandelions
Dulce
Edible Flowers
Eggplant
Fermented Veggies
Garlic
Green Beans
Green Peas
Kale
Kohlrabi
Lettuce
Mushrooms
Mustard Greens
Nightshade Veggies

Onions
Parsnips (high glycemic)
Peas
Peppers
Pumpkin pH 8
Radishes
Rutabaga
Sea Veggies 8.5
Spinach, green 8
Spirulina
Sprouts
Sweet Potatoes
Tomatoes
Watercress pH8.5
Wheat Grass
Wild Greens

ALKALIZING ORIENTAL VEGETABLES
Maitake
Daikon
Dandelion Root
Shitake
Kombu
Reishi
Nori
Umeboshi pH 8.5
Wakame

ALKALIZING FRUITS
Apple pH 8
Apricot pH 8
Avocado pH 8
Banana (high glycemic) pH 8
Berries
Blackberries
Cantaloupe pH 8.5
Sour Cherries
Fresh Coconut
Currants
Dates
Dried Figs

Dried Grapes pH 8.5
Grapefruit pH 8
Guava pH 8
Honeydew Melon
Lemon pH 9
Lime pH 8.5
Mango pH 8.5
Muskmelons
Nectarine pH 8
Orange P
Papaya pH 8.5
Peach
Pear pH 8
Pineapple pH 8.5
Raisins pH 8.5
Raspberries
Rhubarb
Strawberries
Tangerine
Tomato
Tropical Fruits
Umeboshi Plums
Watermelon pH 9

ALKALIZING PROTEIN
Almonds
Chestnuts
Flax seeds
Millet
Pumpkin seeds
Squash seeds
Sunflower seeds
Tempeh (fermented)
Tofu (fermented)
Whey Protein Powder
Yogurt

ALKALIZING SWEETENERS
Stevia
Maple Syrup
Rice Syrup

Raw honey
Raw Sugar (cane)

ALKALIZING SPICES AND SEASONINGS
Cinnamon
Curry
Ginger
Mustard
Chili Pepper
Sea Salt
Miso
Tamari
All Herbs **

ALKALIZING MINERALS
Baking Soda pH 9
Calcium pH 12
Cesium pH 14 Iron
Magnesium pH 9
Manganese Potassium pH 14
Sodium pH 14

ALKALIZING OTHER
Apple Cider Vinegar pH 7.5
Bee Pollen
Dandelion Tea
Kombucha
Lecithin Granules
Molasses blackstrap
Organic Milk (unpasteurized)
Probiotic Cultures
Soured Dairy Products
Green Juices
Green Tea
Herbal Tea
Soya sauce
Veggie Juices
Fresh Fruit Juice
Mineral Water
Alkaline Antioxidant Water

FATS AND OILS
Flax
Hemp
Avocado
Olive
Evening Primrose
Borage
Oil Blends (such as Udos Choice)

F = Fluoride
Water—pH of 4
Penta Water Distilled
Purified tap water
Aquafina (made by Pepsi)
Dasani (made by Coke)
Gatorade
Glaceau Fruit
Le Blue
Metro Mint—Pellegrino (made by Nestle)
Perrier (made by Nestle)
Smart Water
Vitamin Water

Water—pH of 4.5
Reverse Osmosis Water
Ice Age Glacial Water

Water—pH of 5
Appalachian Springs
Ice Age
Perrier F .12
Poland Springs (made by Nestle)

Water—pH of 5.5
10 Thousand BC
Crystal Springs
Dannon Spring
Penta
Pure American Water
All of the above bottled waters have an acidic ph, which does not support health waters

Water—pH of 7
Arrowhead F .5
Crystal Geyser
Deep Park (made by Nestle)
Eldorado Springs
Gibraltar Springs
Northern Crystal
Yukon Springs
Volvic F—ND

Water—pH of 7.5
2-O Below pH 7.7
Aquadeco
Biota
Fiji F .26
Naya
Monasee
Utah Mountain pH 7.7
Whole Foods
Zephyrhills (made by Nestle)

Water—pH of 7.9
Berg Ph 7.8
Eden Springs

Water—pH of 8
Canaqua
Cedar Springs
Deep Rock
Evamore
Mountain Light

Water—pH of 10
Filtered Ionized Alkaline you make with your own Water Ionizer.

INDEX

www.ingramcontent.com/pod-product-compliance
Lightning Source LLC
Chambersburg PA
CBHW032002170526
45157CB00002B/513